DYNAMIC STRENGTH TRAINING FOR ATHLETES

DYNAMIC STRENGTH TRAINING FOR ATHLETES

BOYD EPLEY

UNIVERSITY OF NEBRASKA ATHLETIC STRENGTH AND CONDITIONING COACH

wcb
Wm. C. Brown Publishers
Dubuque, Iowa

Cover photo and interior photos
© Dave Finn

Product photos
Courtesy of AMF

All drawings
Alena Lewis

Copyright © 1985 by Wm. C. Brown Publishers. All rights reserved

Library of Congress Catalog Card Number: 85-71438

Book
ISBN 0-697-00591-7

Book/Diskette
ISBN 0-697-00593-3

No part of this publication may be reproduced, stored in a retrieval system, or transmitted, in any form or by any means, electronic, mechanical, photocopying, recording, or otherwise, without the prior written permission of the publisher.

Printed in the United States of America
10 9 8 7 6 5 4 3 2 1

Contents

Preface ix

1   A Message to Your Parents 1
Both Boys and Girls Can Benefit 2
Begin Strength Training at Age Twelve 2
Motivation 2
Goals 3
Guidelines for the Parent 4

2   A Brief History of Strength Training 6
Weightlifting Is Not for Adolescents 7
Soviets Compete Early 7
Strength Training Is for Athletes 8
My First Lifting Experience 8
Lifting Was Taboo for Athletes 8
Mr. America Shows the Way 9

Strength Is Confidence 9
Hard Work Pays Off 10
Strength Training Comes to Nebraska 10
Searching for More Knowledge 12
Strength Training Catches On 13
A New Organization 14
The Nebraska Way 15
New Equipment Line for AMF 16

3 Understanding Your Body 17
Skeletal Muscle Organization 18
Skeletal Muscle Structure 20
Muscle Fiber Energy Production 21
All-or-None Law 24
Slow and Fast Twitch Fibers 25
Adaptations of Strength Training 26
Strength Training for Women 26

4 Selecting Your Equipment 28
Typical Home Gym Versus Recommended Equipment 28
Additional Equipment Considerations 31
Better Individual Benches 34
Equipment for Supplementary Exercises 36

5 Off-Season and In-Season Training 40
Off-Season Training: The Split Routine 40
Overtraining 41
Cycling 41
Recommended Six-Week Split Routine Cycle for Beginners 42
Week One 42
Week Two 42
Week Three 42
Week Four 43
Week Five 43
Week Six 43
Muscle Soreness 43
Record Your Progress 43
Who Is the Strongest? 48
In-Season Training: Strength Maintenance 48

6 What to Do Your First Day 50
Measurements 50
Stretching Routine 52
Four-Minute Stretching Routine 54
Lifting Exercises with a Bar Only 59

7 Monday-Thursday Lifting Exercises 60
Recommended Exercises for the Chest 61
Bench Press 61
Supplementary Exercises for the Bench Press 63
Incline Press 65
Supplementary Exercises for the Incline Press 67
Recommended Exercises for the Legs 69
Squat, Hip Sled, or Lunge 69
Supplementary Exercises for Lower Leg Development 75
Leg Extension 76
Leg Curl 77
Recommended Exercises for the Stomach 79
Incline Sit-Up 79
Supplementary Exercises for the Stomach 80

8 Tuesday-Friday Lifting Exercises 85
Recommended Exercises for the Back 86
Upright Row 86
Supplementary Exercises for Back Development 87
Recommended Exercises for the Shoulders 90
Military Press 90
Supplementary Exercises for the Military Press 91
Lateral Raise 93
Bent-Over Raise 95
Recommended Exercises for the Arms 97
Curl 97
Supplementary Exercises for the Bicep 99
Tricep Extension 101
Supplementary Exercises for the Tricep 102

9 Speed, Power, Agility, and Endurance Drills 105
Improve Your Weak Areas 105
Step #1—Testing 106
Step #2—Evaluation 108
Step #3—Goal Setting 110
Step #4—Your Program 117
Speed 117
Speed Drills 117
Power 123
Power (Plyometric) Drills 123

Agility 126
   Agility Drills 126

Endurance 129
   Aerobic Conditioning for Endurance 129
   Anaerobic Conditioning for Endurance 129

Recommended Six-Week Conditioning Program 131

10   How to Keep Your Body Strong 144

Don't Overeat 144

Don't Smoke 146

Don't Take Drugs or Drink Alcohol 147
   Marijuana 149
   Cocaine 149

Don't Use Steroids 149

Get Sufficient Sleep 150

Conclusion 150

Notes 153
Appendix 155
Glossary 157
Index 161

Preface

As the strength and conditioning coach of a major college athletic program, I have had many parents request guidance on strength training for their sons and daughters. Most people realize that anyone starting a strength program should follow established procedures, especially young athletes, but few people are familiar with what these procedures are.

This book was written to teach young athletes the correct principles of strength training so they can increase their strength to run faster, jump higher, and improve their confidence. Most books that involve lifting weights are for bodybuilders or weight lifters. I want to emphasize that this book presents a program to help young athletes improve performance. It is not a book on weightlifting. It is a strength program presented along with instructions on how to integrate speed and agility drills to be the best athlete possible. This program is intended to be done at home, however it can be done at school or at a health club.

I wish to express my thanks to Julie Anderson, Derek McWilliams, Kathy Snyder and Patrick Thomas for serving as models for the exercise photos; to Dave Finn for taking the interior photographs; to Alena Lewis for the illustrations; to May Schamp for typing; and Pam Dykeman for proofreading. All product photos are courtesy of AMF American. A special thank you to the University of Nebraska Athletic Department for their help in the preparation of this book, however this does not represent an endorsement.

CHAPTER ONE

A Message to Parents

The reason for starting a strength training program is to achieve high athletic ability. Unfortunately, though, there have been many myths surrounding strength training. Throughout the years athletes have been told that lifting weights would make them muscle-bound, slow them down, and throw off their shots. These myths have prevented many athletes from enjoying the benefits of strength training. The fact is there is no faster way for an athlete to improve his or her performance than through a balanced strength training program.

Performance in most athletic events depends on how well the body can move. Muscles control bodily movement by contracting and pulling the limbs from one position to another. The stronger the muscles, the more forceful these contractions are. A strength training program can improve how high the athlete jumps, and how fast he or she runs, by providing greater strength in the muscles, tendons, and ligament structures. A strength training program involves more than just lifting weights; it integrates running, stretching, speed drills, and agility drills. The result is a faster, more flexible, more muscular, more explosive, better-coordinated athlete. Most parents recognize the value of a strength training program and want their young athletes to get involved, but they are not sure how to go about it.

This book provides recommended strength training guidelines that youngsters can follow to become a better athlete.

Both Boys and Girls Can Benefit

Athletes younger than twelve should concentrate on learning and practicing basic movement skills such as throwing, catching, kicking, tumbling, climbing, jumping, and swinging.

After the age of twelve, a properly conducted strength training or weight training program can benefit all children. Increased muscular strength, stronger connective tissues, stronger bones, better protection against injury, improved coordination, and faster speed of movement can be achieved at this age through a properly conducted strength training or weight training program. As Rousseau said, "The weaker the body, the more it commands; the stronger it is, the better it obeys."

Begin Strength Training at Age Twelve

I advocate strength training as an important factor for children, beginning at age twelve. I believe that strong muscles are important because they provide the power behind all body movements and protect youngsters from injury; also, added strength increases joint stability. It should be noted, however, that any lifting program that is begun before puberty produces less muscular strength than if it were started after puberty is reached. One reason for this is that not until the stage of puberty does a youth's system produce the key hormones responsible for muscle growth.

There are many controversial issues involved in determining the right age to begin lifting. The advantages are much greater than the disadvantages, yet there are still questions concerning the effects of early lifting on a child's body, both physically and psychologically. Serious research has only recently been begun, however it is generally agreed that too much too soon can lead to injury.

Even though the reason for starting a strength training program is to improve athletic ability, it should not be the primary goal in the first years of a youngster's training. The program for the first few years should be progressive in nature, with the idea that the young athlete will continue to train into adulthood. Emphasis should be placed on developing discipline by forming a habit of following the prescribed workouts outlined in this book. Bad habits are tough to break as you get older and eventually keep an athlete from reaching maximum potential. Pay special attention to mastering the techniques for each of the various exercises and drills. Supervision of young athletes lifting weights must also be done with the strictest of measures. Don't be afraid to train with your young athlete; you may derive the same benefits yourself.

Motivation

No athlete, no matter how talented, has ever become a champion without a burning desire to succeed or be a winner. This desire is the internal motivation needed to stimulate an athlete to put in the long hours of practice and make the sacrifices needed to succeed. There are also external motivational factors that you can use to help your son or daughter.

Parents are one of the most important sources of motivation for young athletes. The manner in which you supervise has a direct effect on the attitude and training practices of your athlete. The more knowledgeable you appear, the more respect your opinions will receive.

Another point that goes along with the importance of being knowledgeable and informative is being able to demonstrate the exercises and drills. It is always helpful to be able to show your son or daughter how you want something done. Examples help to reinforce learning, and motivate the athletes. This is a point for being in good shape personally, as athletes invariably perceive the program as being more valid if you take part in it yourself.

If you cannot supervise a training session because of a schedule conflict, arrangements should be made for a qualified spotter to be present. If you want your son or daughter to put forth the effort, you must also be personally willing to invest the time necessary to constantly teach, encourage, and supervise.

The time spent with your children during a workout is a very good time to talk to them and help motivate them.

Goals

Ask your youngster to write down his or her own training goals after realistically looking at their personal strengths and weaknesses. The belief is that athletes tend to work harder toward goals that are more personally important than they would for goals you have written for them.

There are three basic types of goals: short-range, intermediate, and long-range. Short-range and intermediate goals are confidence builders. Short-range may involve daily or weekly goals, such as not missing any workouts, or doing all the recommended repetitions on a difficult exercise. Your son or daughter will need these accomplishments to help see progress towards long-range goals. Long-range goals may be to play on the varsity or to be named to an all-state team, etc.

Please keep in mind that the workouts should be fun. Workouts that are too hard to too intense could lead to physical or mental burnout.

Make sure your son or daughter sets challenging but realistic goals. New and higher goals should be set as the old ones are reached.

Goals are an important means of motivation for young athletes. You can help by reminding them to expect to reach their goals, to visualize themselves reaching their goals, and never to lose sight of their long-range goal. Sometimes it helps to offer an incentive, such as a trip to the ice cream parlor, if a significant goal has been reached. Here are some guidelines you can follow to help your young athlete get started in the right direction.

Guidelines for the Parent

1. A parent should supervise each of the lifting workouts until the young athlete can demonstrate responsibility and competence in warming up properly, in using appropriate lifting techniques, sets, reps, and poundage, and in recognizing unsafe lifting practices. Chapter 5 outlines the recommended program; chapter 6 explains how to get started.

2. The parent should require an orientation period that teaches the proper behavior as outlined in this book.

3. A spotter (in some cases, two spotters) is needed to perform these exercises properly. Spotting for a younger child or pre-teenager can be done easily by most parents. But you must know your limitations. When your child begins to press weight that is more than you can handle, ask another person to help—one on each end of the bar—so that two of you together can replace the weight to the rack, if necessary. Consult the descriptions of exercises in chapters 7 and 8. For each exercise, three paragraphs explain the procedure, value, and necessary equipment. If the exercise requires a spotter, a fourth paragraph explains the safety procedures.

4. Be sure the exercise area in your home will allow the exercises to be performed correctly without sacrificing safety procedures.

5. If the athlete has suffered a sport injury and is seeking exercises for rehabilitation, consult a physician or therapist. This book is not intended for the purpose of rehabilitation.

6. Emergency numbers should be conspicuously posted near the telephone in the event of an injury while lifting. Chances are that you'll never need to use this number, but it is a good idea to discuss emergency procedures in the event that they may be needed. It will also help your youngster realize that he or she is undertaking an activity that requires responsible behavior.

7. The exercise area should be carpeted or covered with a high density rubber flooring, such as Tuflex, to prevent slipping on a slick floor.

8. Do not provide your young athlete with defective equipment. Chapter 4 helps you select good equipment.

9. Regularly check your benches, bars, collars, and cables for any damage or excessive wear that might lead to an accident. The collars should be used on the barbell at all times.

10. All bench tops and sit-up mats should be cleaned regularly with disinfectant.

11. A lumbar supportive lifting belt is recommended for young athletes on exercises such as the Squat or Overhead Press. (See chap. 4.)

12. It is a good idea to wear warm, loose-fitting clothes when lifting in order to keep the muscles and joints warm.

13. Parents need to provide good nutritional meals, and serve desserts without refined sugar. Part of being an athlete is eating good food. As you concentrate on providing better meals for your athlete, you'll be eating healthier too.

Caution: Before starting any exercise program that requires a major increase in physical activity, you should consult with your doctor. If your child has a physical handicap, suffers from a prolonged illness, has problems with hypertension, or any circulatory difficulties, you should have him or her checked as well. Actually, all athletes could benefit from regular checkups. Our bodies are like machines, and need to be in good working order to perform well.

CHAPTER TWO

A Brief History of Strength Training

As the Head Strength and Conditioning Coach at the University of Nebraska for the past fifteen years, I have dedicated myself to researching the steps that are necessary for athletes to develop to their full physical potential. Although people were lifting weights over a hundred years ago, strength training for athletes is a concept that has only become a reality within the past few years.

Strength training has done more to change the athletic world than any other factor in the past fifteen years; it increases one's strength, power, flexibility, and muscular endurance. These increases are proven in athletes who jump higher, run faster, and run for longer periods of time.

Weight training is similar to strength training; however, the goal of weight training is an improvement in fitness rather than athletic performance. You might think of a physical education class doing weight training, while a football team does strength training. Strength training integrates such things as speed drills and distance running, along with the lifting program, and is a much more advanced approach than weight training. Strength training terms, such as *split routine* or *cycling* are not part of the general weight training vocabulary. As you can see in chapter 5, these terms can be very important in making you a better athlete.

Weightlifting Is Not for Adolescents

Weightlifting is different from *strength training* or *weight training*. Weightlifting is a sport in which the *lifter* is trying to see how much weight he or she can lift on a certain exercise. Notice that I refer to the lifter and not the *athlete*. This is because people who lift weights competitively are not usually lifting to become better athletes, but to be the best weightlifters they can be. Weightlifting involves two lifts (the snatch, and the clean-and-jerk).

Powerlifting is another sport in which the individual is trying to see how much weight he or she can lift for one repetition, and not necessarily trying to become a better athlete. Powerlifting includes three lifts that are done in a particular order (squat, bench press, and deadlift).

Powerlifting is a much more popular sport in the United States than weightlifting is, even though weightlifting is a competitive Olympic sport. One reason for this may be that weightlifting is much more technical, and requires a coach to teach the techniques, while powerlifting is easier to learn independently.

Soviets Compete Early

Soviet youngsters are allowed to begin lifting competitively at an early age (11–13 years).

What does competitive weightlifting at such a young age do to these Soviet children? The biggest danger voiced by researchers seems to be whether or not such competition will interfere with bone growth. The growth of the bones takes place along the discs of cartilage called the epiphyseal plates, which are located on the inner side of the epiphysis. The extent of bone growth is usually determined genetically, but small adaptations can occur. These adaptations can be caused by a number of things: amount of stress to which the bone is subjected, the nutritional quality of the diet, the amount of injury sustained, and disease. When a lot of stress is applied to a bone, it may show signs of wear, and small portions of the joint cartilage can be chipped off. The epiphysis or the epiphyseal plate, could close at an early age and stop the growth of the bone. Compression to either the epiphysis or epiphyseal plates before closure can retard the growth of the bone structure.

According to Soviet research, however, there is no difference in height between weightlifters and non-weightlifters. This infers that the epiphyseal discs do not undergo any damage that might interfere with normal growth.

Most U.S. researchers believe that a child should not weightlift or powerlift competitively until at least age seventeen. They contend that before puberty a youngster grows too fast, and that competitive lifting may damage physical growth and contribute to the development of high blood pressure. Before puberty the joints are not prepared for the stress of heavy weightlifting or powerlifting; after puberty the joints are much stronger and can stand up better to the demands of competitive lifting. I don't think competitive lifting of any kind is the direction to take in becoming an athlete. Football players at the University of Nebraska are not allowed to participate in lifting competitions.

Strength Training Is for Athletes

Strength is only one of the important components that is beneficial to a successful athlete. The acquisition of speed, power, and agility are actually more important to an athlete than strength. Since strength is the easiest component to develop, youngsters often get too caught up in gaining strength and, consequently, overlook the other aspects of training. A balanced strength and conditioning program helps develop each of the major components of athletic success. Chapter 9 shows you how to integrate both types of drills into a plan of action.

My First Lifting Experience

My first experience with a set of barbells proves the need for guidelines for young athletes who wish to start exercising with weights. In the remainder of this chapter, I provide the details of that first experience, and show you how strength training has changed my life.

In 1957, when I was in fifth grade, doctors determined that I had asthma and advised my parents to move with me from Nebraska to Phoenix, Arizona. While walking to school my first day in Phoenix, I met a classmate named Danny Lundberg. After a few weeks of school, he invited another boy named Ronnie and me over to his house. Danny took us out to his garage, where his older brother kept a set of weights. This was my introduction to weightlifting, and it is probably not uncommon to many other youngsters' first experience. The bar had seventy-five pounds on it at the time, and Danny was eager to demonstrate how he could clean this bar first to his chest, and then over his head—like they did on television in the Olympics.

Without benefit of stretching, warming up with a lighter weight, or learning proper lifting technique, I gave it a try, too. Peer pressure can be very strong at age ten. I'm sure you have heard the expression, "I dare you." It wasn't easy, but I managed to lift the bar overhead and return it to the floor, much to Danny's approval. Next it was Ronnie's turn. Ronnie wasn't the athletic type, and I was worried for him because I knew how hard the lift had been for me. Ronnie managed to lift the bar to his chest, but when he jerked it overhead he lost control of the bar. He fell over backward, and the bar nearly landed on his head. It didn't take us long to realize that there was some technique involved with the sport of weightlifting, and that lifting should not be done without knowing the proper procedures.

Lifting Was Taboo for Athletes

My next experience with weightlifting came in seventh grade when my parents surprised me with my own 110-pound barbell set. The barbell set came with instructions, but they were based entirely on competitive weightlifting techniques, including the snatch, the clean-and-jerk, and the overhead press (which has since been discontinued as a competitive lift). There were no instructions on how to improve athletic performance, and I didn't realize then that coaches did not recommend lifting weights for this purpose. There was no such thing

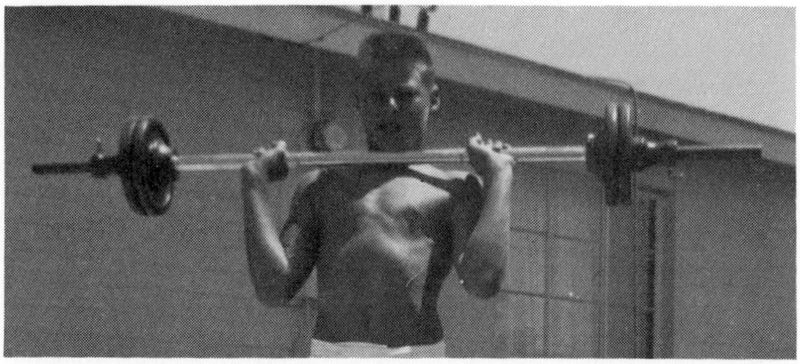

Figure 2.1
Young Boyd Epley with First Set of Weights

as strength training for athletes. After the novelty of my new barbell set wore off, it began collecting dust. It wasn't until the summer after my junior year in high school that I gave another thought to the weights.

Mr. America Shows the Way

That summer (1964) I became friends with a fellow my age named Pat Neve, who had a set of dumbbells at home. He was a bodybuilder who eventually became Mr. America and Mr. U.S.A. Pat did arm exercises almost every time a commercial came on TV, and I was surprised at the dedication he showed to lifting weights. He was very serious about his exercise routine, and would even drag me along to another friend's house to train with him. His friend, Ken Cole, was a teacher/coach at a grade school in our part of town, and had a sophisticated set of equipment in his backyard where he let weightlifters and bodybuilders train. I learned that bodybuilding was a form of competition in which the participants don't actually see how much weight they can lift, but are judged for muscular development, symmetry, and presentation during a series of poses called a *posing routine*. I noticed that these bodybuilders trained much differently than weightlifters did. They did a variety of exercises to develop each muscle, rather than concentrating on perfecting their form to see how much weight they could lift on a particular exercise. They also used lighter poundages, but repeated each exercise more times than the weightlifters did.

I wasn't really interested in competitive weightlifting or bodybuilding, but I was interested in getting stronger for football. Rather than impose on Pat's friend, I joined a health club so that I could work out regularly. During that summer I combined some of the bodybuilding and weightlifting concepts with my own ideas and integrated some running drills to prepare for my senior football season.

Strength Is Confidence

My progress that summer seemed more dramatic than it would be for someone beginning a strength and conditioning program today, because at that point in time very few athletes were lifting weights. It was like being the only person in town who had watered his lawn the entire summer. My lawn was noticeably greener and healthier than all the others.

During my junior year football season, I had not taken practice very seriously. In fact, I had been known to play "tag" or "touch-me-last" during practice. Consequently, I did not play in even one varsity football game during my junior year, although as the backup quarterback I weighed 160 pounds. When I reported back for football that fall for my senior season I weighed 180 pounds. The coaches and other players had trouble recognizing the new me. These twenty additional pounds were in the form of bigger muscles—something very uncommon to high school athletes at that time.

What did bigger muscles and added strength mean to me? In one word, it meant "confidence." Lifting weights that summer started a chain of events that completely changed my life. The purpose of this book is to point out how you, too, can realize the benefits of what I call *strength training*. My physical progress caused me to be more and more disciplined and dedicated to my schedule. I became serious about anything that would help me to be a better athlete. I watched what I ate, went to bed early, and tried not to miss any workouts; I was hooked on strength training and anxious to show the results. I can still remember the first day of football practice my senior year. Because of the physical development I had achieved over the summer, the coaches moved me to linebacker. Much to the surprise of everyone, with my new confidence, my new strength, and my new determination, I was able to set a new school record for most tackles and was named the Outstanding Defensive Player of the Year.

Hard Work Pays Off

The hard work had paid off, but it was only the beginning. I continued to lift weights, and used this new strength to set records as a pole vaulter. I managed to add the Outstanding Track Man Award to my honors. However, I broke my leg pole vaulting just before the state championships. This was a very disappointing injury because it not only kept me out of the state meet, but also excluded me from scholarship recognition. I saw this as just another obstacle I would have to overcome, so the next year I directed my energies to pole vaulting at Phoenix Junior College. The strength training really paid off when I earned a scholarship to the University of Nebraska after placing second in the National Junior College Pole Vault Championships.

Strength Training Comes to Nebraska

When I left Arizona in 1967 after ten years, I had outgrown my asthma problem and had picked up a basic knowledge of weightlifting and bodybuilding. I knew how to convert the principles of each area into strength training to improve athletic performance. Until I went into the weight room at the University of Nebraska I didn't realize that I had any special knowledge or that I would quickly be considered "the expert on strength training."

Huge football players wandered into the weight room with no idea of how to train, and not one of them could bench press three-hundred pounds. A few of them noticed the exercises that I was doing and began asking me questions on how they might train. I had put in several

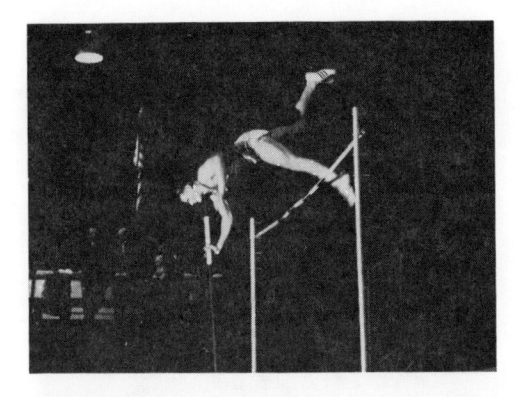

Figure 2.2
Boyd Epley sets New Nebraska School Record

years of strength training, so even though I was only a 180-pound pole vaulter, I was much stronger than any of the football players.

The extra strength enabled me to set school vaulting records for Nebraska, but it wasn't until a back injury during my senior year in 1969 that strength training took over as my main goal in life. The injury forced my retirement from vaulting, and led me to spend even more time in the weight room. More and more of the football players were asking for my help. One day Dr. Tom Osborne, the Football Assistant Coach (now the Head Coach), called me into his office to ask me if I was the one who was showing the football players how to lift weights in the weight room. I wasn't sure whether to say yes or no. At that time lifting weights was not recommended by any football coaches in the country. Nebraska athletes had no stretching program, no winter strength or conditioning program, no summer strength program, no testing of strength, agility, or power, and no lifting during the season. I said, "Yes, I am the one who has been helping some of your players get stronger." He said he had noticed definite improvement in their performance, and wondered if I could help the other players as well. Boy, was I relieved.

I told him that the weight room was not large enough to handle very many players at one time, and it would need more space in addition to more equipment. He asked me to make a list of what we would need, and he bought everything on the list. I made another

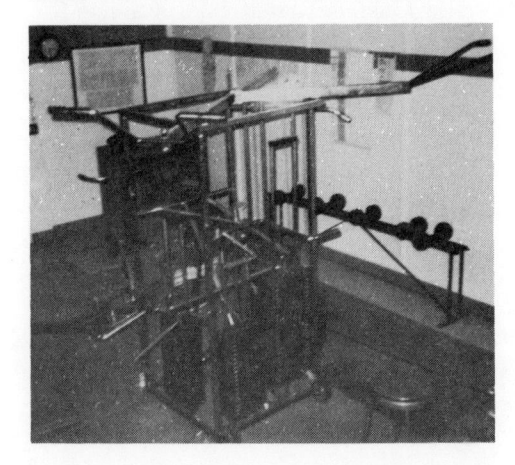

Figure 2.3
The Beginning. The Nebraska weight room in 1967.

A Brief History of Strength Training 11

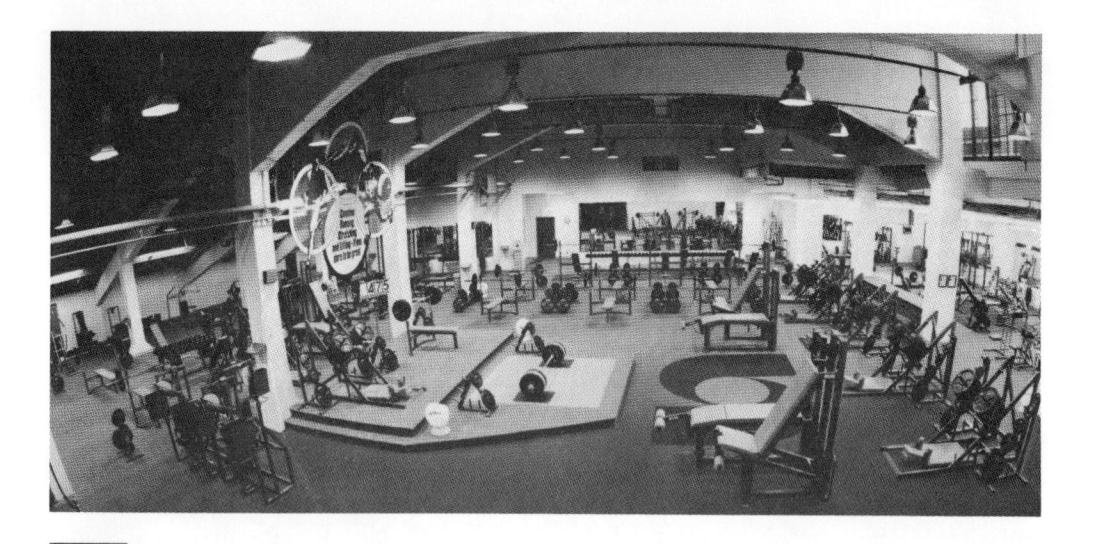

Figure 2.4
The Nebraska Strength Complex

list, and he bought everything on that list, too. I've been making lists ever since, and the University of Nebraska now has the largest football strength training facility in the world, in addition to several weight rooms for other sports.

Searching for More Knowledge

It didn't take Coach Osborne long to realize the potential in strength training for helping athletes to develop themselves physically. He asked me to instigate a program for all players on a year-round basis, which meant lifting weights during the competitive season. This was unheard of in athletics in 1970, so I set out to learn all I could about strength training for athletes. Unfortunately there wasn't much information available. As I worked on my master's degree, I asked the instructors if I could gear my coursework toward learning more about strength training programs and facilities for athletes. They were extremely cooperative, and adapted most of my projects so that they would relate to my needs. Between 1970 and 1972, as I worked on these master's degree classes, I also entered physique, powerlifting, and weightlifting competitions to learn everything I could about gaining maximum strength and muscle growth. I took a powdered protein supplement that helped my body weight jump from 180 pounds to 234 pounds. I was surprised at the early success I enjoyed in these competitions, and I organized both a weightlifting team and a powerlifting team for the University, and brought weightlifting meets to Lincoln, Nebraska for the first time. I seemed to have a natural ability for lifting competitively, and winning came very easily.

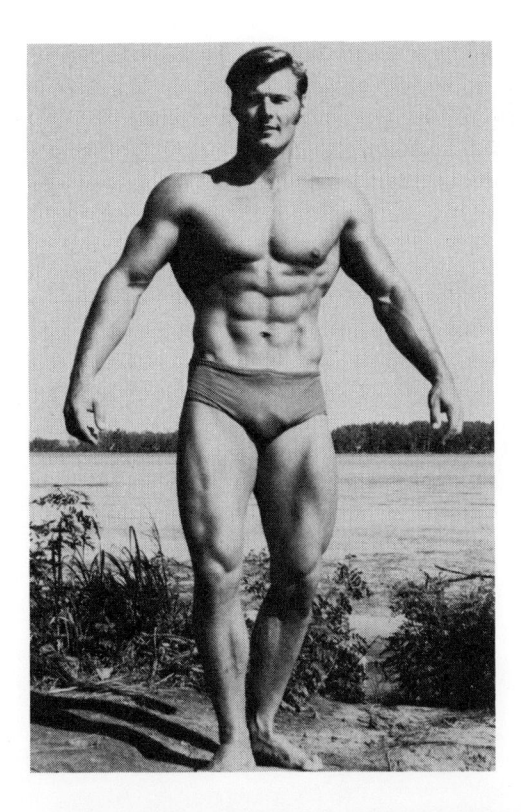

Figure 2.5
Boyd Epley—The Competitor

The 1972 Midwestern A.A.U. Outstanding Lifter Award was presented to me by Mabel Rader, the Chairperson of the Midwestern A.A.U. She said:

> This year Boyd Epley established eight Nebraska state records and five Midwestern records in lifting, as well as winning the physique titles of Mr. Nebraska, Mr. Midwestern and Mr. Mid-America. He has qualified this year for the A.A.U. Class I patch in all three—weightlifting, powerlifting, and physique competition. This is really a great accomplishment, since it is seldom that a man is outstanding in both, and never in all three.

Strength Training Catches On

I retired from any further competition after 1972 because my goal during this period wasn't to compete, but rather to transfer any knowledge I could gain from the competitive lifting circles to developing a strength training program for the University athletes to improve performance. I had visions of a lifting program that could benefit athletes. Asking the entire football team to lift weights back then was about like driving a car the wrong way down a one-way street, but being strong myself certainly helped get all the players going in the right direction. My strength training program caught on very quickly after the players were re-tested in the 40-yard dash and realized that the strength training program had increased their speed.

With the strength program for football players well under way, my next effort was to help the other sports, which included women's athletics, until all fourteen sports at the University had strength programs. It didn't take long for other universities to notice the progress Nebraska athletes had made. With back-to-back National Championships and impressive victories (over Alabama 38–6 and over Notre Dame 40–6) in football, it wasn't long before coaches were copying the Nebraska strength program and asking to hire my assistants to start a strength training program for them.

The following is a list of teams since 1974 that either currently have or at one time hired one of my assistants.

Universities	*Professional Teams*
Arizona State	Cleveland Browns
Arkansas	Detroit Lions
Clemson	Houston Oilers
Florida	L.A. Express
Iowa State	Minnesota Vikings
Kansas State	New York Giants
Miami	New York Jets
Missouri	New York Yankees
Notre Dame	San Francisco Giants
Ohio State	
Oklahoma	
Oregon	
Southern Methodist	
Stanford	
Texas A & M	
UCLA	
University of Nevada–Las Vegas	
Washington State	
Wyoming	

A New Organization

Although I sent out one-thousand letters with invitations to NFL teams, colleges, strength equipment companies, and the larger high schools from states surrounding Nebraska, only seventy-six people showed up in Lincoln, July 28, 1978, but from this first meeting emerged a new organization called the National Strength and Conditioning Association (NSCA). They elected me president and chairman of the board of directors in each of the first five years. The board is made up of regional directors from across the nation. The national office was my desk for the first three years, but is now located at 251 Capitol Beach Boulevard, Lincoln, Nebraska 68508. The *NSCA Journal* was developed to provide coaches and athletes with information on strength training methods and procedures. The focus of the *Journal* is

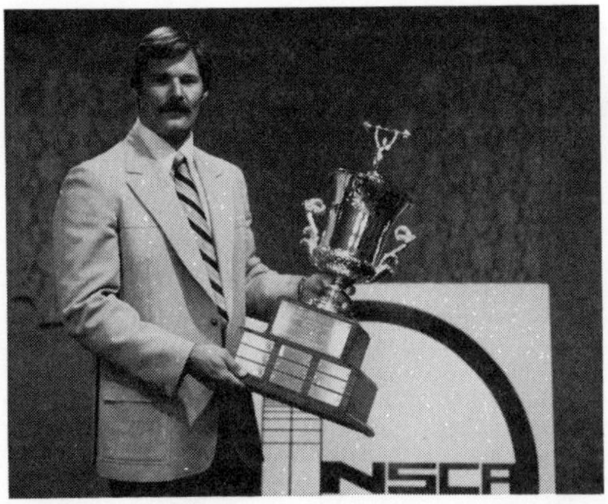

Figure 2.6
Boyd Epley—America's first
Strength Coach of the Year

on strength training information. The *Journal* discusses the basic components of conditioning: strength, speed, power, cardiovascular endurance, muscular endurance, flexibility, and agility. Each component receives extensive coverage in order to provide well-balanced, total conditioning specific to an individual sport. Weightlifting and powerlifting articles are not included. Interest has been tremendous as the NSCA has grown to over eight-thousand-five-hundred members, including twenty-seven foreign countries. Nearly 50 percent of the membership are senior high and junior high school coaches. Some of its activities include a committee that has been developed to establish scholarships for young strength coaches, and a research committee that works to bridge the gap between the strength coach and the sport science research laboratory. The NSCA also communicates to members through regional, state, and local workshops. Over sixty NSCA-sanctioned clinics are held each year. Once each year the Association sponsors a national convention where a Strength Coach of the Year Award is presented.

The Nebraska Way

In 1979 I received permission from the University of Nebraska to form a private consulting corporation in an attempt to give more individual help to coaches and athletes nationwide. This consulting service (Body Enterprises) has had a big impact on strength and conditioning in this country, serving athletes with programs we call "The Nebraska Way." In one year alone over one-thousand-two-hundred schools took advantage of these consulting services. The products and services cover a wide range—from everything a beginner would need at home to the most sophisticated programs in the NFL—including computer software.

New Equipment Line for AMF

In 1980 AMF (American Manufacturing Foundry) asked me to design and endorse a line of strength and conditioning products for athletes. AMF is a huge corporation with annual revenues of over five billion dollars. My first design was the hip sled for leg development. I wanted a machine that could work the legs safely without spotters. I was really excited when

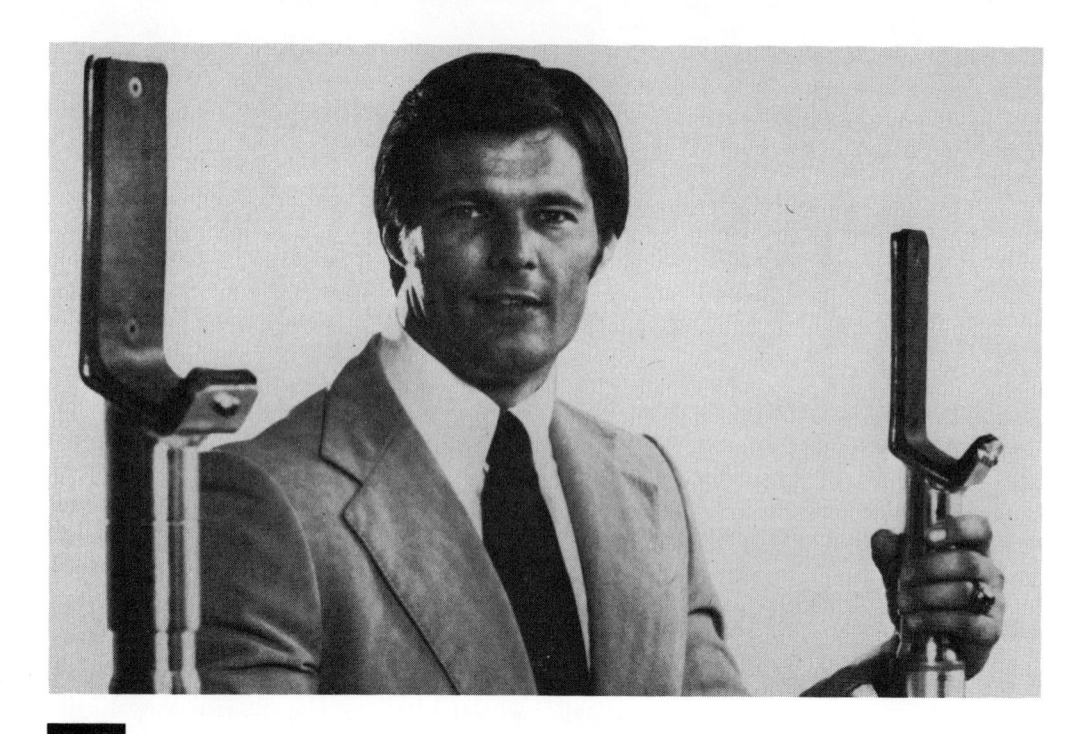

Figure 2.7
Epley has designed a full line of strength and conditioning equipment for AMF.

Joe Gitch, the National Sales Manager for AMF American, called and asked me to fly to their plant to evaluate the first prototype hip sled. Back then they were calling it the EPR–150. EPR stood for Epley Power Rack; 150 was how much the carriage weighed. I asked for a few modifications in the prototype before it was shipped to Lincoln for the football players to test.

The hip sled met with very rapid success, not only for Nebraska players, but nationwide. The next few years led to the development of an entire line of AMF strength and conditioning products, which have spread to athletes worldwide.

It is evident that strength training has meant a great deal to me. I have dedicated my life to providing instruction for coaches and athletes in order to enable them to share in the tremendous rewards that strength training can offer. Most of this information has been geared to high school, college, and professional coaches and athletes. But, hopefully, this book will offer it to you, too, so you won't have any bad experiences while lifting weights for the first time, like Ronnie and I had back in Danny Lundberg's garage.

CHAPTER THREE

Understanding Your Body

Your body is made up of over six-hundred muscles, and they account for one-half of your total body weight. The primary function of your muscles is to contract (shorten in length) in order to produce movement of your body parts.

Understanding how the body produces movement might be made easier by comparing the body's nervous, muscular, and skeletal systems to the accelerator, engine, and transmission of an automobile. When the accelerator pedal is depressed, a signal is sent to the engine, and power is generated. The transmission sends this power out to the wheels to produce movement of the car.

This sequence is similar in the body. Your brain sends a signal to your muscle by way of a nerve. The muscle responds by contracting and generating power. Since your muscle is attached to your bone by tendons, the muscle-tendon-bone connection produces movement at the joints.

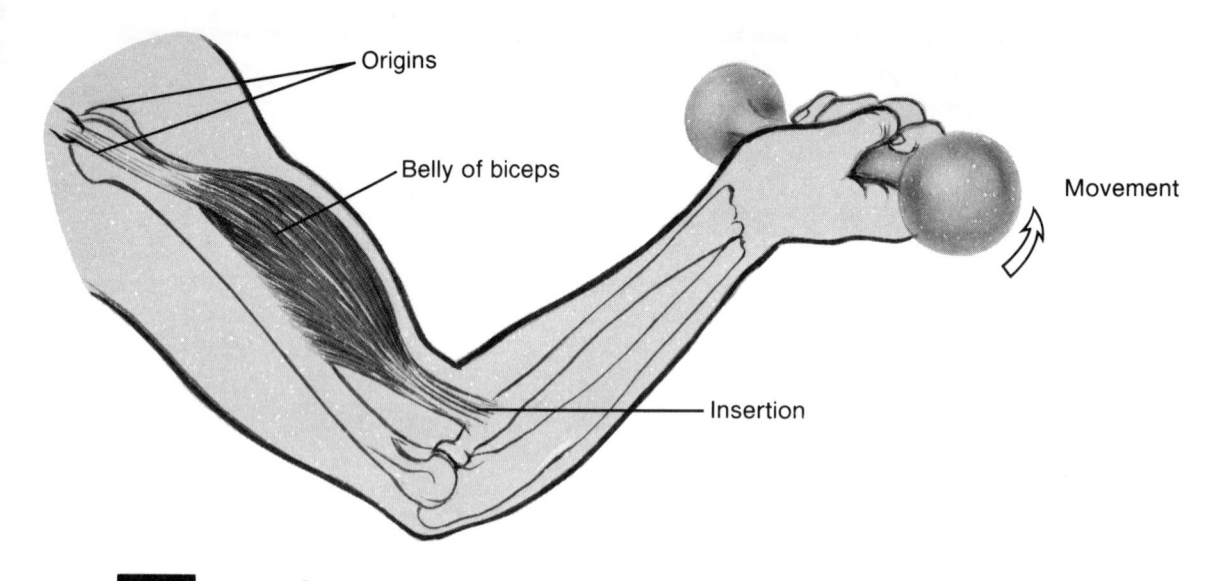

Figure 3.1
Bicep Anatomy

Skeletal Muscle Organization

If I asked you to make a muscle, you would probably respond by flexing your bicep, the muscle on the front part of your upper arm. The bicep has a thick middle part, known as the *belly* of the muscle. It forms what we call the *peak* of your bicep, and tapers at the ends to form tendons. These tendons attach to your bones, then act as levers for the muscles. The tendon attachment at one end of your muscle is referred to as the *origin,* and at the other end as the *insertion.* The origin of the bicep attaches to the shoulder bone, while the insertion of the bicep goes past the elbow and attaches on the forearm bone (fig. 3.1). The forearm is moved toward the origin by flexing the bicep muscle.

Your bicep can only pull the forearm toward the shoulder; it cannot push the forearm back to its original position. In fact, all of your muscles cause movement by pulling. The muscles do not push, as you might think they do. The bicep teams up with the tricep muscle, which is the muscle on the back of the upper arm, to return your arm to the starting position. When the bicep contracts, the tricep muscle must relax to allow the bicep to work. To straighten the arm back again, the tricep muscle contracts pulling the forearm back to its original position, and the bicep must relax (fig. 3.2).

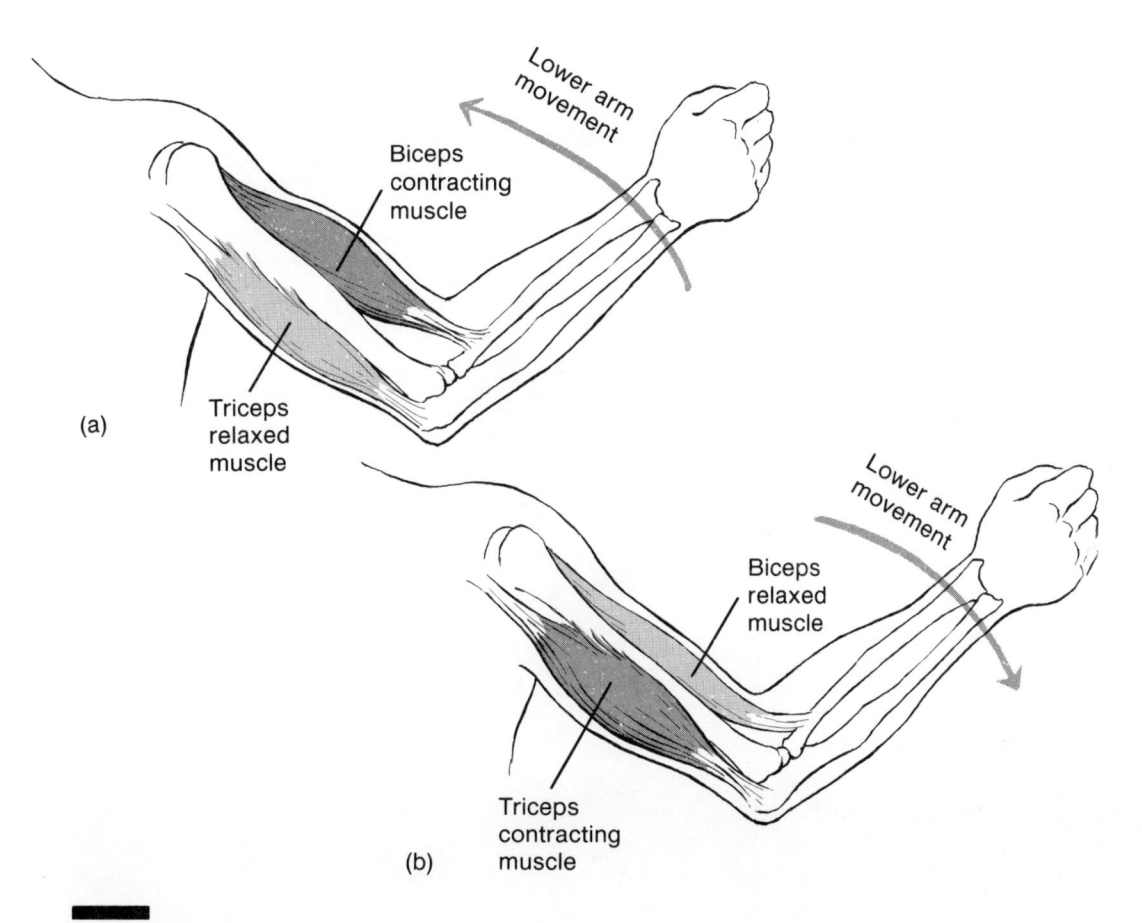

Figure 3.2
(a) Bicep flexion
(b) Tricep extension

Most of the body is arranged so there are muscles on both sides of a joint. A joint is where two bones come together and work like door hinges so movement can occur. All muscles work in pairs, one flexing, or pulling in toward the body; the other extending, or pulling away from the body. It is important that your strength program includes exercises that work both sides of a joint, or both muscles that work as a pair, and not just one of them.

Some other common muscle groups that work in pairs are the thighs (front of leg) and hamstrings (back of leg), as well as the chest and back muscles. A balanced program includes at least one exercise for each major muscle group in your body (figs. 3.3 and 3.4).

Chest (Pectoralis)

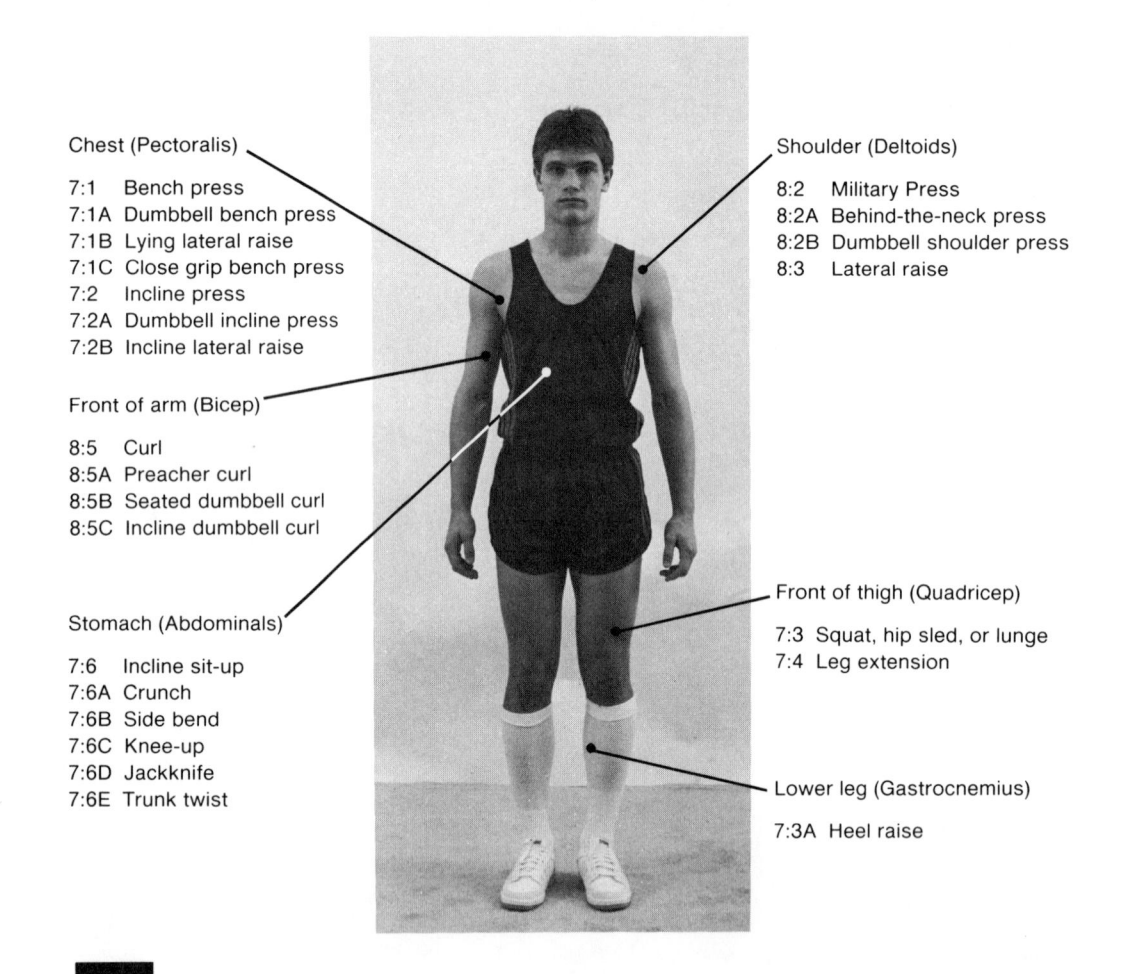

7:1   Bench press
7:1A Dumbbell bench press
7:1B Lying lateral raise
7:1C Close grip bench press
7:2   Incline press
7:2A Dumbbell incline press
7:2B Incline lateral raise

Front of arm (Bicep)

8:5   Curl
8:5A Preacher curl
8:5B Seated dumbbell curl
8:5C Incline dumbbell curl

Stomach (Abdominals)

7:6   Incline sit-up
7:6A Crunch
7:6B Side bend
7:6C Knee-up
7:6D Jackknife
7:6E Trunk twist

Shoulder (Deltoids)

8:2   Military Press
8:2A Behind-the-neck press
8:2B Dumbbell shoulder press
8:3   Lateral raise

Front of thigh (Quadricep)

7:3   Squat, hip sled, or lunge
7:4   Leg extension

Lower leg (Gastrocnemius)

7:3A Heel raise

Figure 3.3
Anatomy Chart—Front

Skeletal Muscle Structure

Each of your muscles is made up of bundles of muscle fibers called fasciculi. These bundles contain various numbers of muscle fibers. A single muscle fiber is composed of many individual muscle fibrils (fig. 3.5). These fibrils are composed of smaller parts called filaments, which are made up of protein. Thick filaments (myosin) and thin filaments (actin) lie parallel to each other, as shown in figure 3.6. Study this figure closely. Each segment is enlarged so you can see the structure of your muscles.

Upper back (Trapezius)

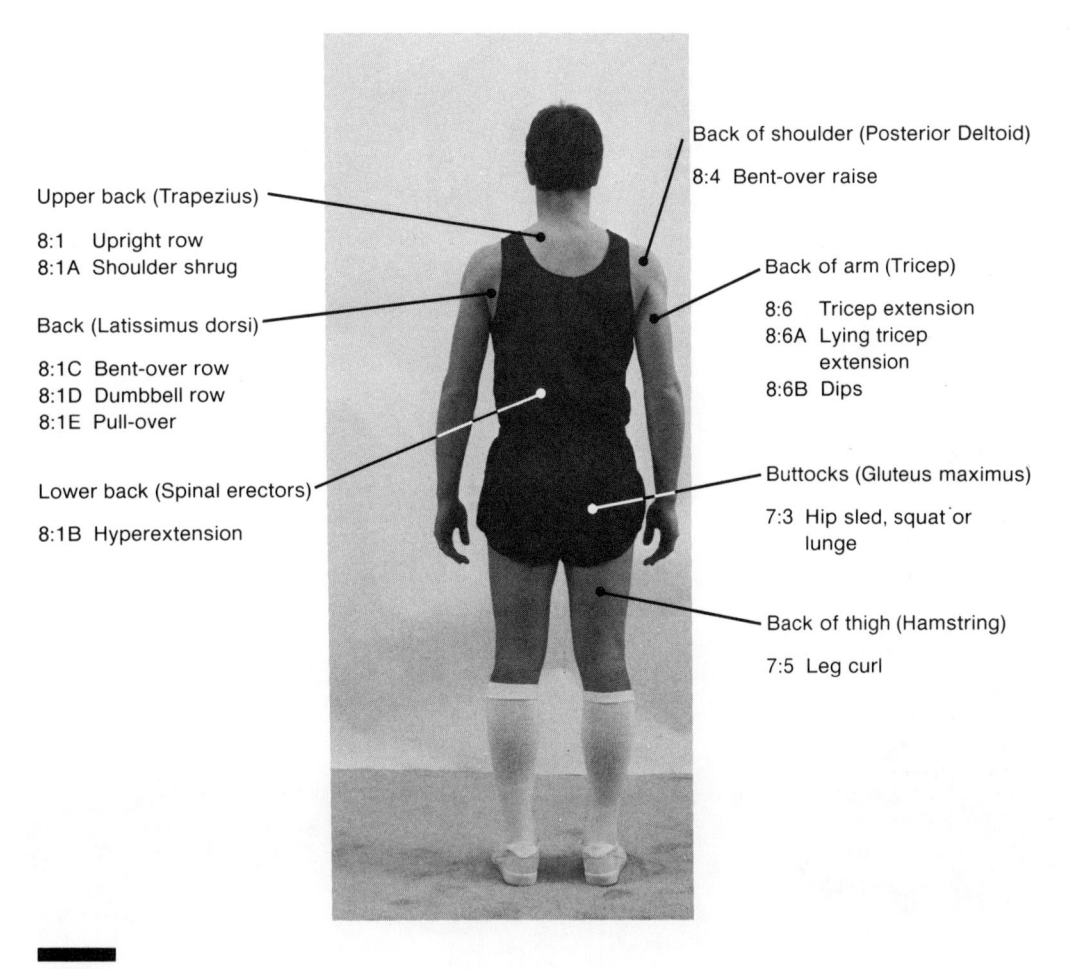

8:1   Upright row
8:1A Shoulder shrug

Back (Latissimus dorsi)

8:1C Bent-over row
8:1D Dumbbell row
8:1E Pull-over

Lower back (Spinal erectors)

8:1B Hyperextension

Back of shoulder (Posterior Deltoid)
8:4 Bent-over raise

Back of arm (Tricep)

8:6   Tricep extension
8:6A Lying tricep extension
8:6B Dips

Buttocks (Gluteus maximus)

7:3 Hip sled, squat or lunge

Back of thigh (Hamstring)

7:5 Leg curl

Figure 3.4
Anatomy Chart—Back

Muscle Fiber Energy Production

Capillaries are small blood vessels that deliver oxygen and energy-rich foods to your muscle fibers. The food then goes through a series of chemical reactions to produce what is called adenosine triphosphate (ATP). ATP is the energy fuel used by your body to contract its muscles in the same way an automobile uses gasoline to accelerate. The energy released from ATP pulls the actin filaments along the stationary myosin filaments, causing the muscle to shorten and contract (fig. 3.7).

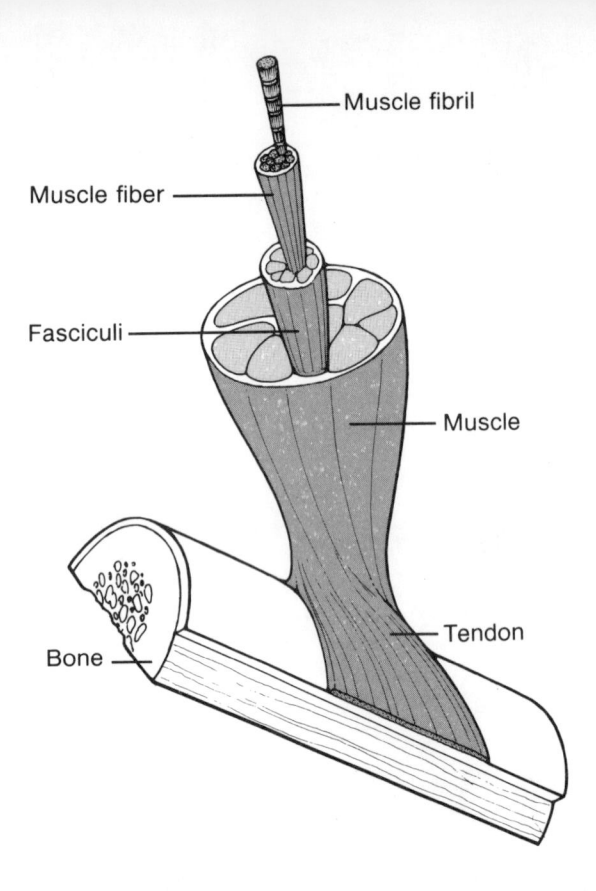

Figure 3.5
Skeletal Muscle Structure

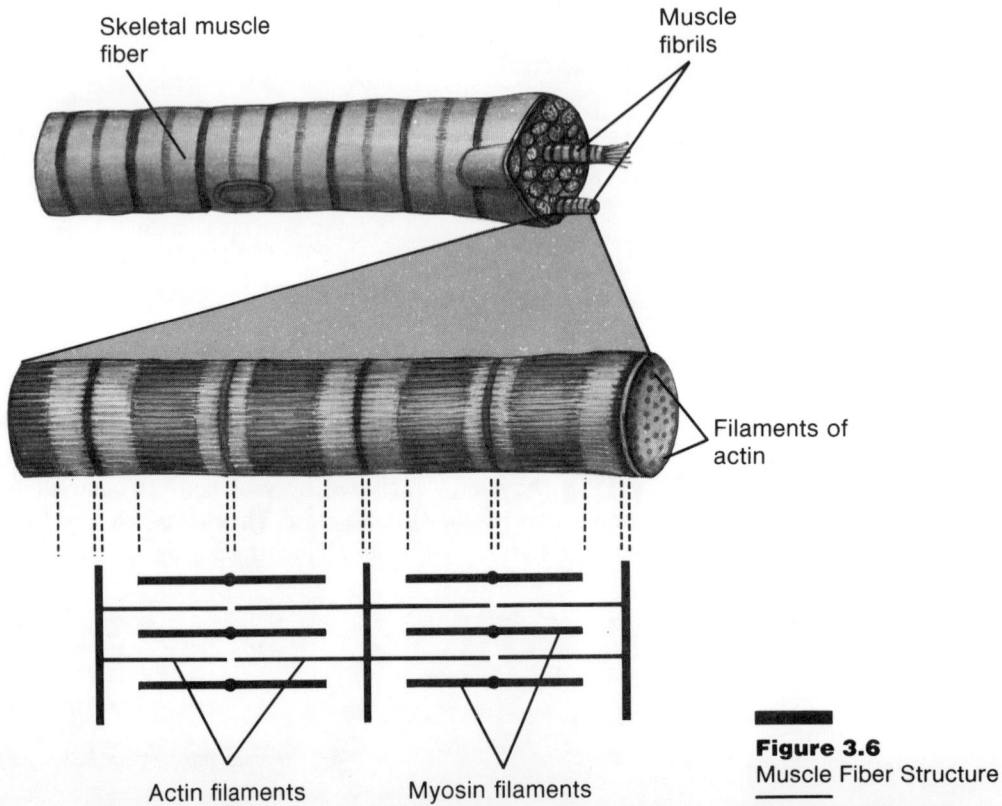

Figure 3.6
Muscle Fiber Structure

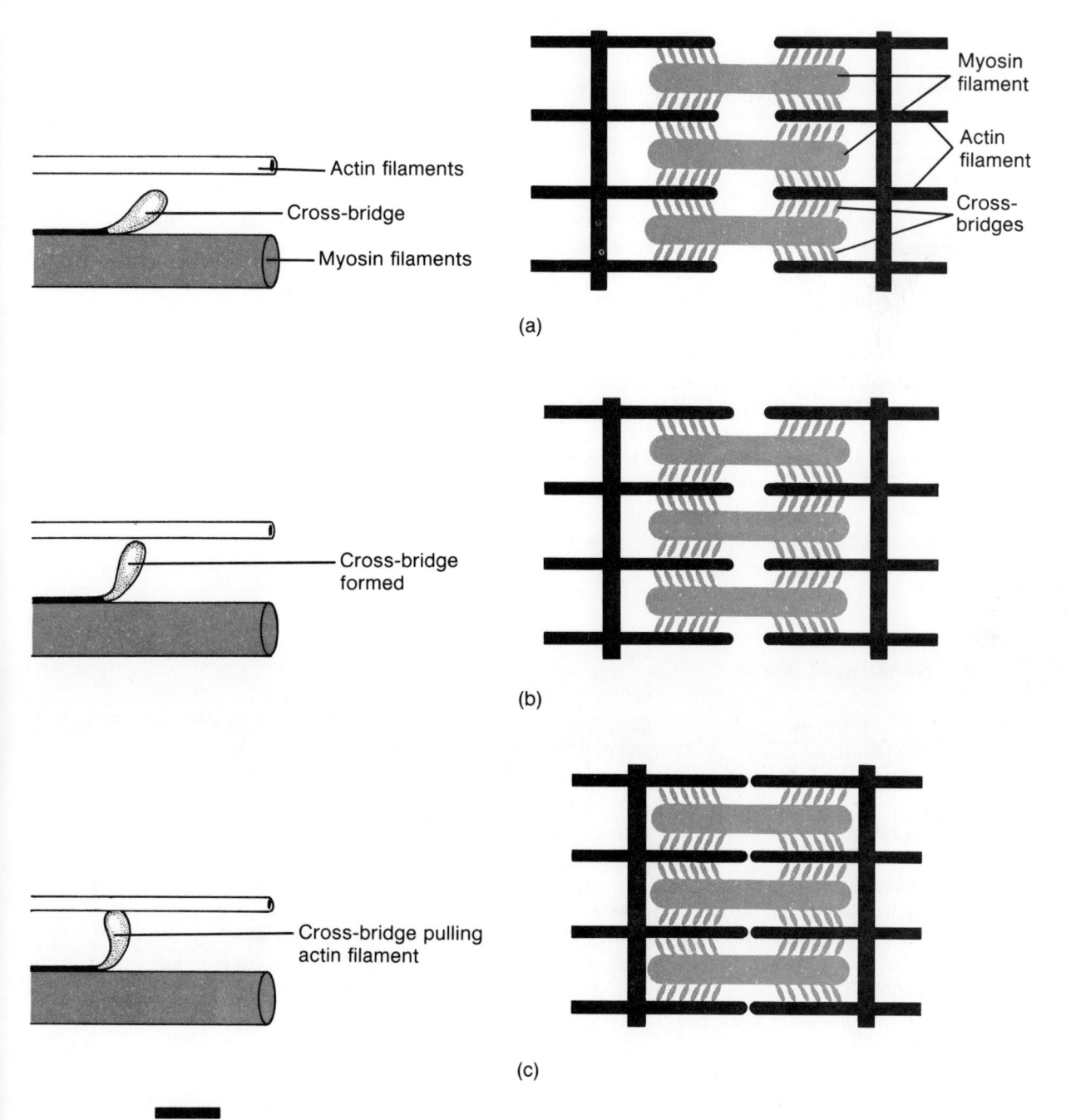

Figure 3.7
Summary of Muscle Contractions

Understanding Your Body 23

ATP energy that uses oxygen is called *aerobic exercise*. An example of this type of exercise occurs when you run, swim, walk, or bike at a pace that can be continued for five minutes or longer. At first your normal breathing will bring in enough oxygen for the exercise, but as your exercise speed increases you breathe more rapidly. This causes more oxygen to be used, and increases the amount of ATP that must be supplied so your muscles can continue to contract.

Your muscles can only store small amounts of this ATP fuel at any one time. When you exercise at short, intense distances (like back-to-back 40-yard dashes), you cannot breathe fast enough to provide enough oxygen to your muscles. Since oxygen is necessary to supply more ATP, you can only run a few full-speed, back-to-back 40-yard dashes before you run out of ATP fuel. This kind of ATP utilization without oxygen is called *anaerobic exercise*. Your ATP could be restored in a matter of minutes if your muscles were allowed to rest.

During strength training you are exercising anaerobically, or without oxygen. A set usually lasts only fifteen to thirty seconds, then you feel a burning sensation in your muscles. This is caused by something called lactic acid, which is a waste product of ATP. When lactic acid buildup becomes too great, it causes your muscles to become fatigued to the point where you can no longer contract them. This is why rest periods are necessary between sets. During this recovery time the body goes through a series of chemical reactions to supply more ATP. The amount of rest needed between your lifting sets is dependent on how intense your exercise period has been, and also whether you want to increase strength or endurance. You should rest one to two minutes between each set for strength gains, but only ten to twenty seconds between sets if your goal is to improve your endurance.

All-or-None Law

A motor unit is made up of a motor nerve and the group of muscle fibers that it attaches to (fig. 3.8). When a motor unit is stimulated, it will either contract fully or not at all. All contractions are of the same intensity because a muscle cannot contract harder at one time than at another time. Muscles are made up of many motor units, and in a relaxed muscle very few motor units are active. Just enough are stimulated at any one time to keep the body from collapsing. This is known as muscle tone. To lift a weight it is necessary for more motor units to become active so the muscle can contract. This is known as motor unit recruitment.

The number of motor units that are activated is related to the amount of weight you are lifting, or the amount of weight you *think* you are lifting. Lifting a light weight takes very few motor units. The greater amount of weight you lift, the greater the number of motor units activated. This is why it is so important that you concentrate mentally while lifting. Your brain can call on more muscle fibers to contract if you concentrate on what you are doing.

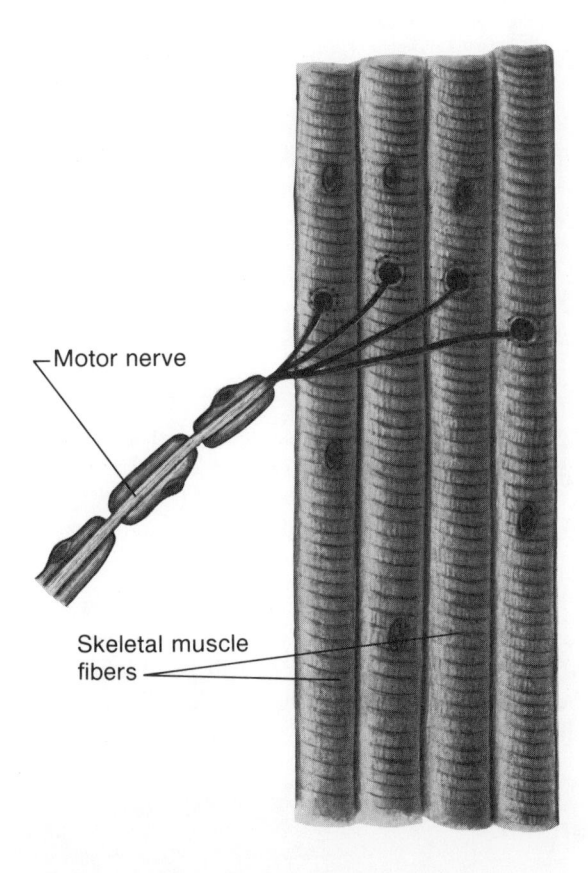

Figure 3.8
Motor Unit

Slow and Fast Twitch Fibers

There are two types of muscle fibers: slow twitch for endurance, and fast twitch for speed. Everybody has a certain combination of slow and fast twitch fibers, which is determined at birth. A person with a greater percentage of slow twitch fibers can excel at endurance-type activities, such as distance running and swimming. A person with a high percentage of fast twitch fibers can succeed at sprinting and power-type athletics such as football, basketball, and baseball.

Your strength training program will help you recruit more of your fast twitch (speed) fibers, but will not increase the number of these fibers. The speed fibers are able to contract faster and more powerfully than slow twitch fibers, also they increase in size and diameter to a greater extent than slow twitch fibers as a result of your strength training. The larger speed fibers will enable you to lift heavier weights. Distance runners don't have large muscles because they are recruiting slow twitch muscle fibers when they run.

Adaptations of Strength Training

Muscular strength is developed only when you use the overload principle. To overload your muscle means to work it beyond normal. The muscle responds by adapting to the work imposed. Following is a summary of the adaptations that will take place as a result of your strength training program.

1. Increase in number of motor units activated
2. Increase in size of muscle fibers, especially the fast twitch type
3. Slight increase in capillary density
4. Increase in strength of tendons
5. Increase in density of bone at tendon attachment sites
6. Ability of muscles to store more ATP for energy production
7. Ability of muscles to tolerate lactic acid buildup

Your muscles, and only your muscles, can produce movement of your body, so when you improve muscle strength your movements become more efficient. You will be able to run faster and jump higher, and you'll look better and feel better about yourself. This extra confidence will carry over into your everyday life.

Strength Training for Women

In sports involving speed, strength, and endurance, men generally excel over women. The lower strength levels of women when compared to men is reflective of the difference in body size and body composition. This is the primary reason for the difference in athletic performance between men and women. At the age of ten, performance levels are about equal because body size and strength differences are minimal prior to puberty, but during puberty these differences begin to widen and become fully developed in adulthood.

On the average, women are about four inches shorter and thirty pounds lighter than men. Women also tend to carry about 10 percent more body fat, which means that an average man's body composition consists of much more muscle in relation to fat than an average woman's body. Because of the greater muscle size and percentage of muscle, most men are much stronger than most women. In fact, women possess about two-thirds the strength of men.

Women do not have the same capabilities to increase muscular size as men. This is because a hormone called testosterone, which contributes to muscular size, is present in quantities ten times greater in the normal male than in the normal female. Even though men have greater capabilities to increase in muscular size, women tend to lose more fat than men as a result of strength training.

When comparing women to men, you must consider the muscle groups being compared. While women are much weaker in the chest, shoulders, and arms, they compare more equally in leg and hip strength. If only lean body mass is considered, (total body weight minus fat weight), women are almost equal in strength per unit of lean body mass. Some studies have shown that women have slightly greater leg strength per unit of lean body mass.

Even though women are smaller and don't have the same ability to increase muscular size that men do, the female has the same potential for strength development as does a male of comparable size. The quality of muscle in both female and male in terms of its ability to exert force is the same. There is no need to devise special strength programs for females because the same programs can be equally effective for both men and women.

CHAPTER FOUR

Selecting Your Equipment

One of the most common questions I am asked by young athletes is, "Should I exercise at home or should I join a health club?"

The answer to this question is simple. The majority of health clubs have Nautilus, Universal, Paramount, Hydra-Gym, or similar machines that are made for adults. Children will not fit into many of these machines properly, therefore health clubs are usually not the answer for young athletes. Unless a health club has barbells and dumbbells (and most of them don't), the young athlete must train at school or purchase home exercise equipment.

When selecting home exercise equipment you should keep in mind that your equipment must be sturdy enough to support not only the weight you are lifting, but also your body weight. Your equipment should also be sturdy enough so that, as you get older and stronger, it will still be capable of handling the heavier poundages that you will use.

Typical Home Gym Versus Recommended Equipment

Figure 4.1 is a typical home gym. I generally recommend that young athletes do their strength training at school, because a typical home gym like this does not provide for a balanced program of safe exercises. Schools usually provide sturdier and safer equipment, as well as supervision during lifting. These factors eliminate my biggest concerns with lifting at home.

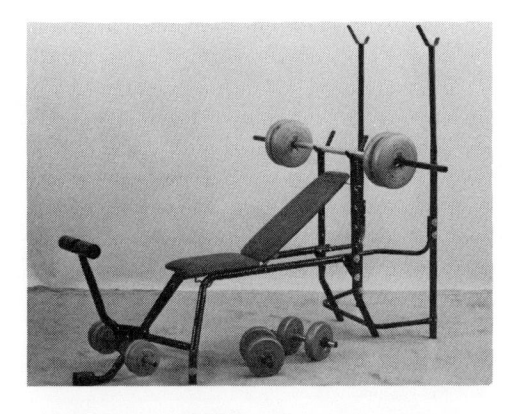

Figure 4.1
Typical Home Gym. Includes a bench that adjusts from a flat bench to an incline bench of 45 degrees. The bench also has a leg extension and leg curl attachment on the front, and a squat rack in the back. The barbell set is plastic, and includes a pair of dumbbells.

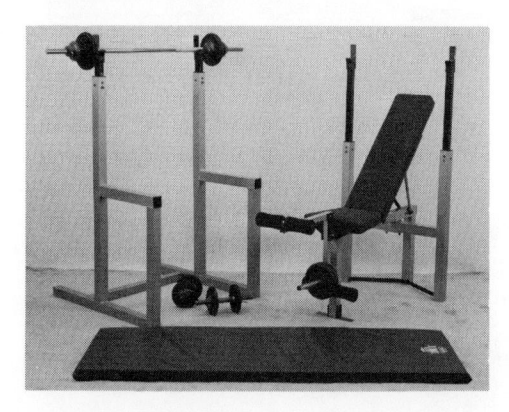

Figure 4.2
Recommended Equipment for Your Home Gym. 1.) Bench press bench (Body Enterprises #460–400). 2.) Squat cage (Body Enterprises #460–800). 3.) 110-pound iron barbell set. This set includes a pair of 14-inch adjustable dumbbells. 4.) Home exercise mat (AMF 45–100) 2'×6'×2".

According to the Consumer Product Safety Commission, half of all lifting injuries occur in ten to nineteen year olds, and more than half of these injuries occur in the home.[1] If you have quality equipment and use the proper technique, you should not experience injuries from lifting. In fact, just the opposite is true; a lifting program actually helps prevent injuries.

Figure 4.2 is the basic equipment that I recommend for your home gym. The equipment in the typical home gym and the equipment in the recommended home gym may look similar, but they are not comparable at all in terms of safety. Let's take a closer look.

The typical home gym equipment does not provide for adequate leg development. It is uncommon to see a squat cage in the home; therefore, good leg development at home is also rare. A squat cage is recommended so you can squat inside the rack safely, and in the event that you cannot stand up with the weight, the barbell will come to rest on the lower level, thus preventing a possibly hazardous situation. See chapter 7 for instructions on the squat exercise.

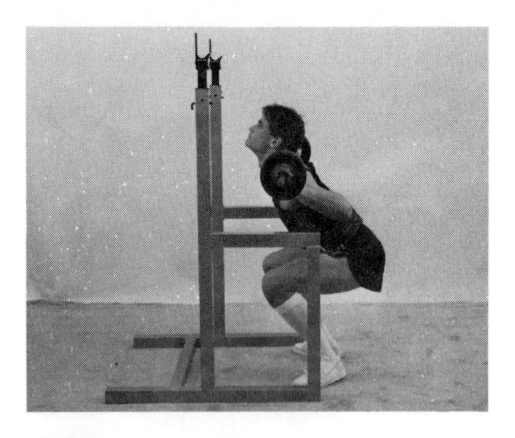

Figure 4.3
Squat Cage. The squat cage prevents possible hazardous situations.

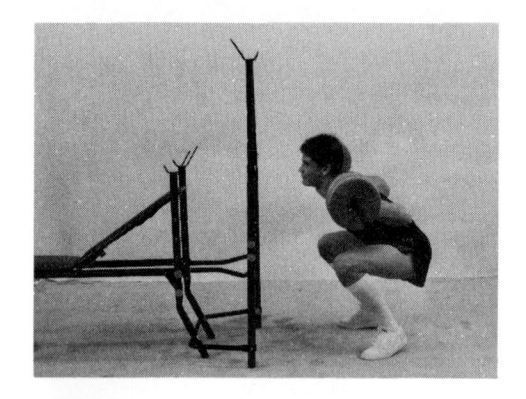

Figure 4.4
Squat Uprights. Squat uprights do not provide safety when doing squats.

The typical home gym may have squat uprights on the back of the bench for you to rest the bar on between sets, however these do not provide any safety for you in the event that you cannot stand up with the weight. When using squat uprights, two or three spotters are required, but they aren't usually available in the home gym. If you can't do squats safely at home, don't do them at all. A squat cage for your home can correct this problem. One can be constructed out of wood or metal.

The bench press bench is also much safer with a lower level; however, most do not have a safety level for the bench or incline. If your bench press bench does not have a safety level, you should not do bench presses or incline presses without a spotter to assist you with putting the bar back on the rack. If you are lifting alone you should use dumbbells to do the bench press or incline press exercise.

The typical home gym does not include a mat for stretching or sit-ups either. A two inch thick home exercise mat measuring two ft. by 6 ft. works well for both stretching exercises and stomach work. Advanced athletes may want to add more difficulty to their sit-ups by providing an AMF Inclined Sit-Up Board (No. 436–040) and Ladder (No. 436–041).

Plastic weights are preferred by some families, but I'm not sure why. Possibly they fear dropping an iron barbell would result in damage to their carpet. If you are lifting correctly you are not going to be dropping any weight on the floor. Iron plates are actually better for the young athlete for two reasons:

1. It is difficult to get very many of the plastic plates on a five-foot bar because of their width. (Be sure to get a solid bar and not a hollow one.)

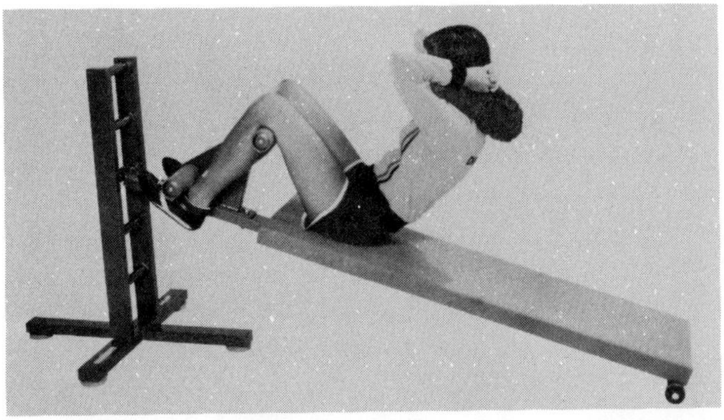

Figure 4.5
Incline Sit-Up

2. As you get older and stronger, you'll need to add more plates to your 110-pound set. Twenty-five pound iron plates can be purchased from almost any sporting goods store to beef up your beginner set. Advanced athletes usually purchase a 6-foot long standard bar and collars for use on the bench press and squat exercises where heavy weights are used, then they use their old 5-foot bar for arm work.

Some advanced athletes think they need to purchase an Olympic set, but I really don't think that is necessary for the home gym. Olympic sets are very expensive; their only real advantage over the standard bar is that the Olympic bar revolves. The plates are not interchangeable, as the standard plates have a 1⅛-inch hole while the Olympic plates have a 2-inch hole.

Additional Equipment Considerations

The recommended home gym equipment provides for the majority of the exercises presented in this book; however, if you have the space and can afford to add to your home gym equipment, there are several additional items that will improve your program. Your program of exercises is dependent upon your lifting facility, so any improvement in your exercise equipment also brings about an improvement in your lifting program. Any of the items described in this book can be purchased from Body Enterprises, P.O. Box 80517, Lincoln, NE 68501, unless a specific address is listed.

We said earlier in this chapter that the squat cage makes leg development safe for home use. The items in figures 4.6 to 4.10 can make your squat cage even safer.

Squat Stool
The squat stool (fig. 4.6) adjusts in height to allow you to squat to the depth of your choice. It also provides a T-shaped base that permits use with a heel board or in a regular flat-footed squat.

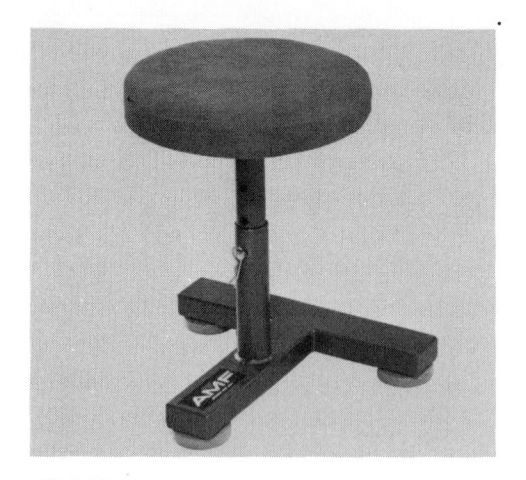

Figure 4.6
Squat Stool

Figure 4.7
Heel Board

Heel Board
Most young athletes will want to use a heel board (fig. 4.7) when doing the squat because of tightness in the back of the heel.

Lifting Belt
A leather belt (fig. 4.8) provides support for your lower back. Some experts say the belt is not necessary, but athletes tell me they feel they can lift ten to fifteen pounds more with the belt on because it gives them confidence and a sense of security. I recommend using a belt for the squat and the shoulder press exercise, and for any other exercises you choose. Belts are usually one-hundred-millimeter wide (approximately four inches), and can be purchased from almost any sporting goods store for $20–$30. Advanced athletes sometimes spend up to $100 on a lifting belt for features such as colored suede coverings, a variety of thicknesses ranging from seven to thirteen-millimeter, and chrome buckles.

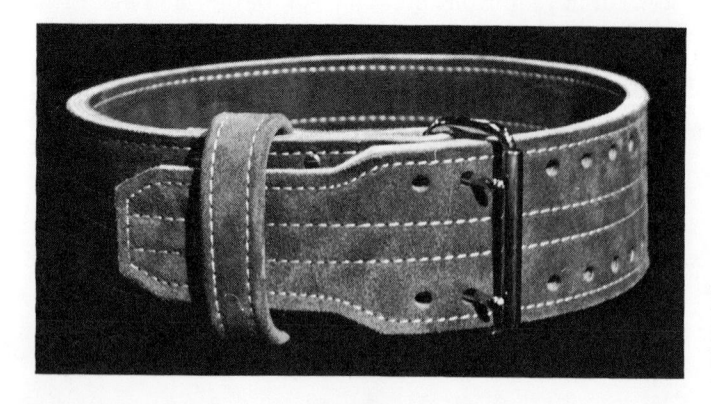

Figure 4.8
Lifting Belt

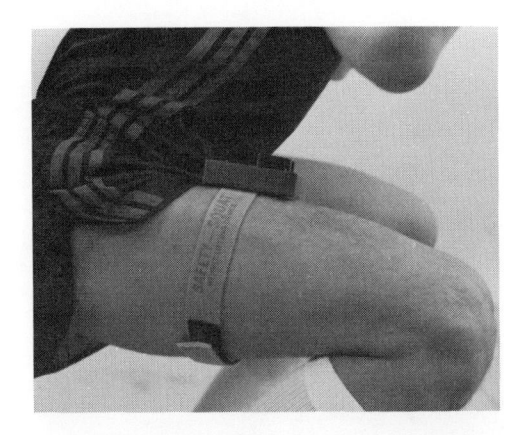

Figure 4.9
Safety Squat

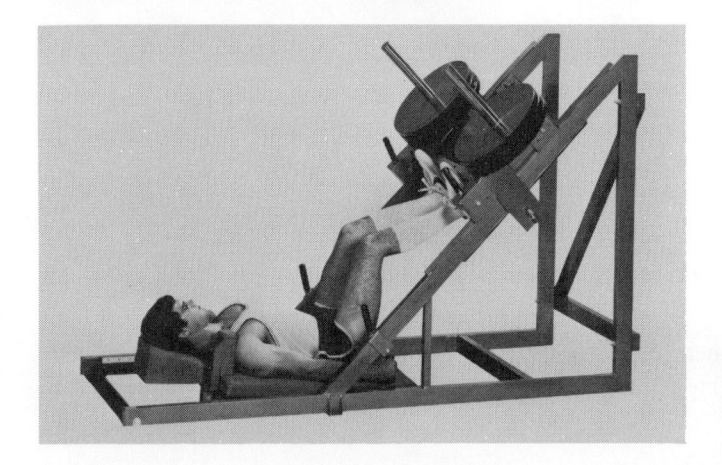

Figure 4.10
Hip Sled

A brochure on lifting belts can be obtained from Power Place Products, Inc., 124 East State Street, West Lafayette, IN 47906.

Safety Squat
A new device, called the Safety Squat (fig. 4.9), is designed for persons who want to know when they have reached a depth of parallel. The device "beeps" when your thigh reaches a position parallel with the floor. The safety squat can be purchased from Safety Squat, Inc., Route 1 Alebia Dr., East Prairie, MO 63845.

Hip Sled
The AMF Hip Sled (fig. 4.10) is a safer method of leg development than the squat. This machine is for persons five to seven feet tall. The hip sled eliminates the need for spotters or lifting belts, because it greatly reduces the stress on your lower back. While this may be one of the safest ways to work your legs, not everyone can afford the luxury of a hip sled (No. 436–003) in their home.

Selecting Your Equipment

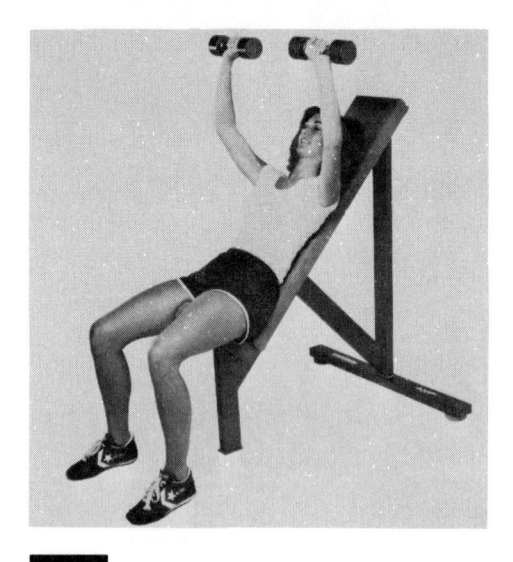

Figure 4.11
Seated Incline Bench

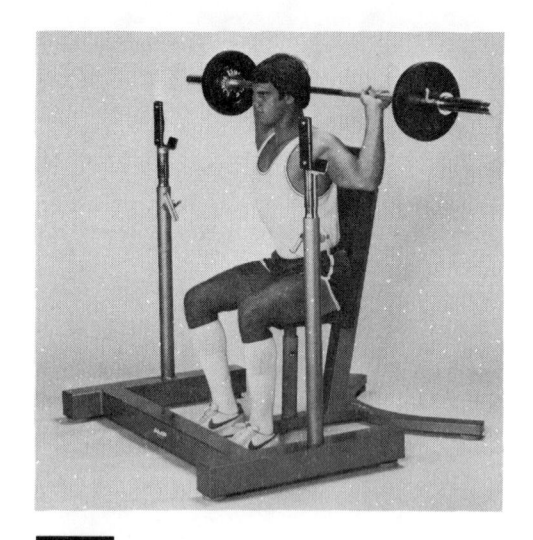

Figure 4.12
Shoulder Press Seat

Better Individual Benches

Seated Incline Bench
The AMF Seated Incline Bench (No. 436–032) (fig. 4.11) is usually used with dumbbells for chest and arm work. Having a fixed incline eliminates the need to adjust your bench to an incline position each time.

Shoulder Press Seat
The AMF Shoulder Press Seat (No. 436–350) (fig. 4.12) provides support for your back during the exercise. It also adjusts for the different heights of individuals. When you do the shoulder press while sitting on your bench press bench, you don't have quite the stability that you would with the shoulder press seat. The added support allows you to handle heavier poundages.

Preacher Curl Bench
The AMF Preacher Curl Bench (No. 436–037) (fig. 4.13) allows your arm to be stabilized so the development is directed to the front of your arm (the bicep).

Work Bench
The AMF Work Bench (No. 436–033) (fig. 4.14) is a handy, multi-purpose bench used for a variety of seated and lying exercises. Your bench press bench could provide for these exercises also.

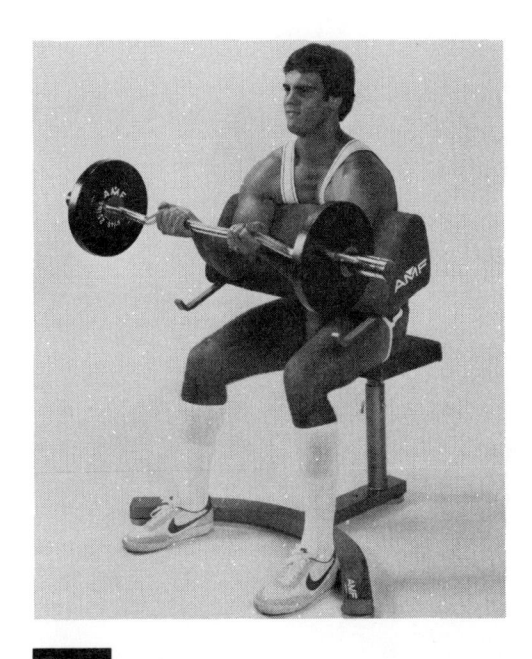

Figure 4.13
Preacher Curl

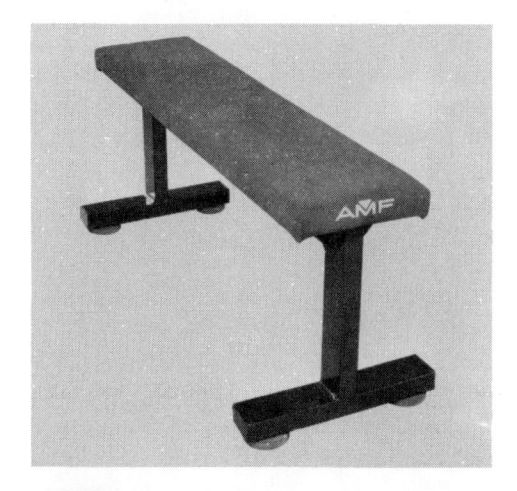

Figure 4.14
Work Bench

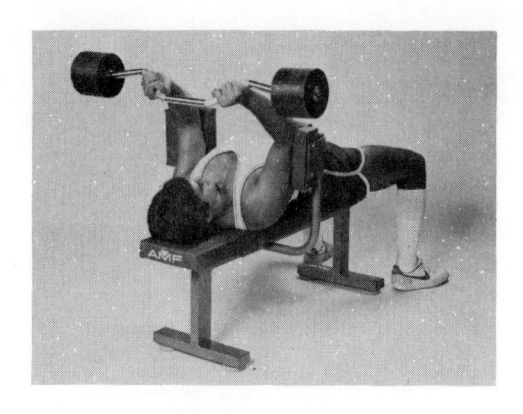

Figure 4.15
Tricep Bench

Tricep Bench

The AMF Tricep Bench (No. 436–340) (fig. 4.15), like the preacher curl bench, allows your arm to be isolated. Development is directed to the back of your arm (the tricep). It is actually a work bench with an adapter to isolate your arms. The bar catch for the bar to rest on between sets is not pictured.

Selecting Your Equipment   35

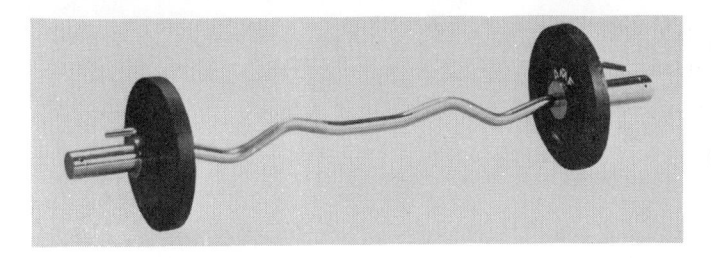

Figure 4.16
E-Z Curl Bar

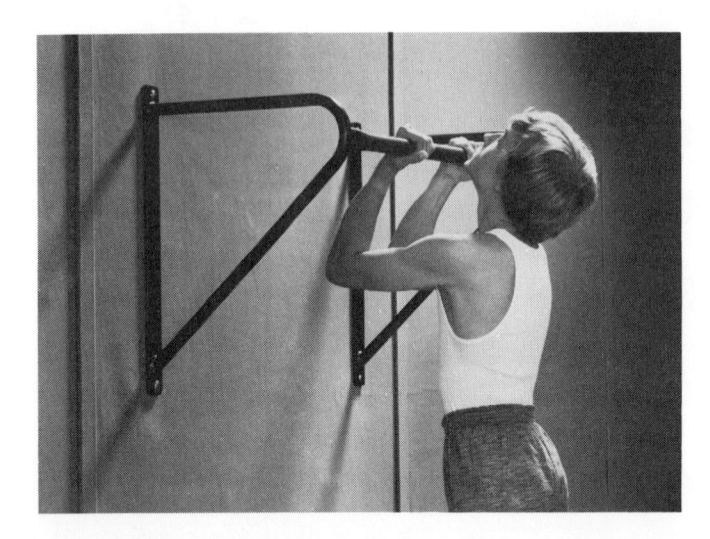

Figure 4.17
Pull-Up Bar

Equipment for Supplementary Exercises

E-Z Curl Bar
Some athletes prefer the bent angle of the AMF E-Z Curl Bar (No. 436–221) (fig. 4.16) rather than the straight bar. The angled bar puts less stress on your wrist. However, using the straight bar for curls will tax the upper inside portion of your arm to a greater degree.

Pull-Up Bar
Pull-ups are a positive way to develop your back muscles. The AMF Pull-Up Bar (No. 409–003) (fig. 4.17) can be mounted to the wall.

Dumbbells and Rack
For athletes who can afford the luxury of AMF Dumbbell Sets (fig. 4.18), they come in four sets, five to twenty-five pounds (No. 436–267), thirty to fifty pounds (No. 436–268), fifty-five to seventy-five pounds (No. 436–295), and eighty to one-hundred pounds (No. 436–296). A rack is required for each set (single, No. 436–210; double, No. 436–209). Dumbbells can also be ordered in separate pairs. You should be able to adjust the weights on your pair of dumbbells without the expense of a fixed set of dumbbells. It takes a little extra effort but with proper budgeting of time it can be done.

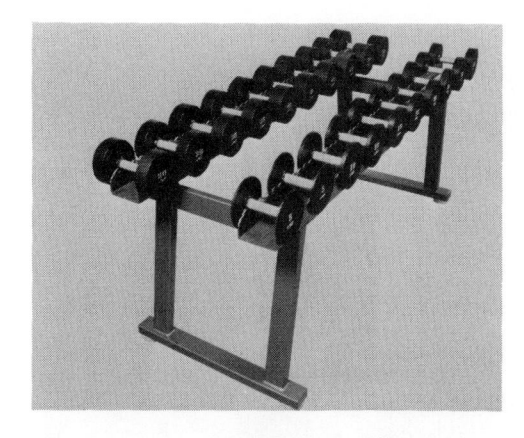

Figure 4.18
Dumbbells and Rack

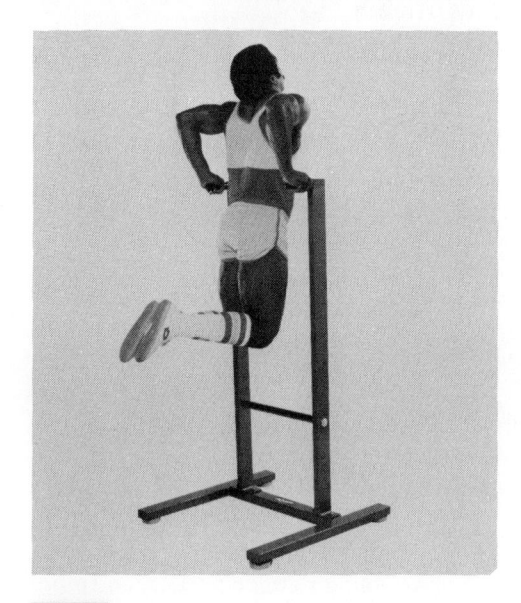

Figure 4.19
Dip Stand

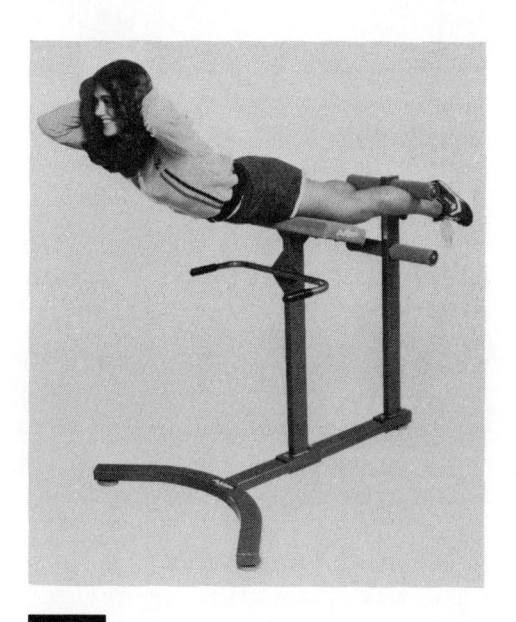

Figure 4.20
Hyperextension Bench

Dip Stand
This AMF Portable Dip Stand (No. 436–042) (fig. 4.19) would be a nice addition to anyone's home gym. Dips are a good way to develop the back of your arm (tricep).

Hyperextension Bench
The hyperextension exercise develops the erectors of your lower back. To perform this exercise properly, you will need a hyperextension bench (fig. 4.20). (AMF No. 436–036)

Figure 4.21
Lifting Gloves

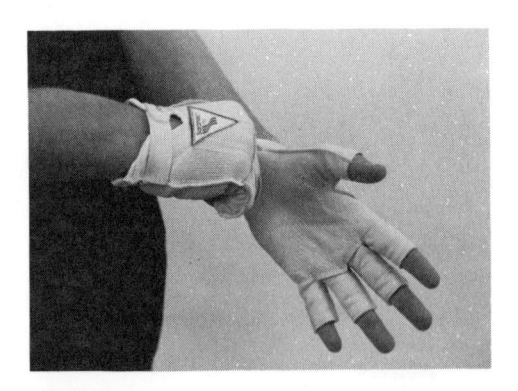

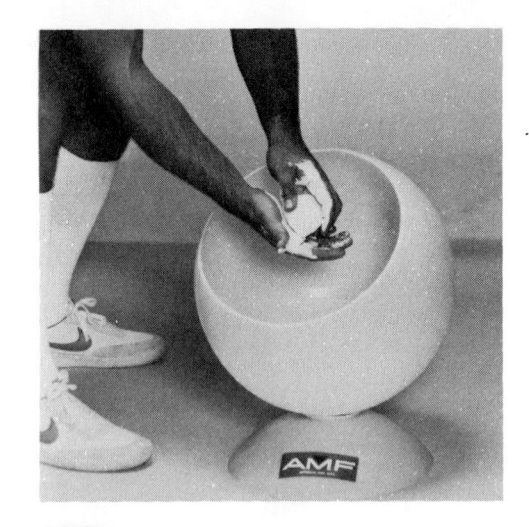

Figure 4.22
Chalk

Lifting Gloves
Lifting gloves (fig. 4.21) have become popular to provide a good grip on the bar, and to prevent build-up of callus on the palms. If they cannot be found at your local sporting goods store, try your bicycle shop.

Chalk
Chalk (fig. 4.22) will keep your hands dry, and provide a good grip on the bar, without gloves. Chalk can be purchased from most sporting goods stores. (The chalk bowl is AMF No. 407–011.)

Broomstick and Jumprope
A broomstick (fig. 4.23) can serve as a tool for stretching, and also to help warm up before lifting.

A jumprope should be used at the conclusion of your workout. A good jumprope can be purchased at a local sporting goods store, and should be part of your exercise equipment.

Specific Programs
Strength training programs specific to the needs of a particular sport (fig. 4.24) are available from Body Enterprises, P.O. Box 80577, Lincoln, NE 68501.

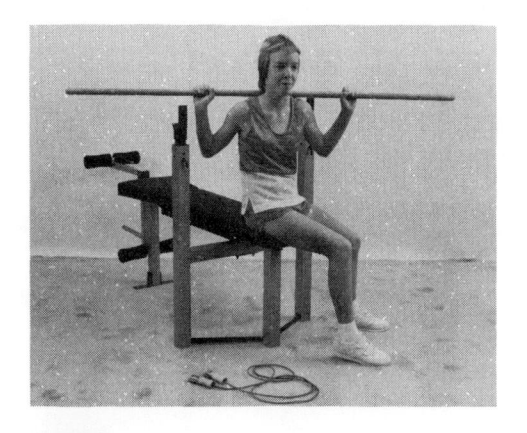

Figure 4.23
Broomstick and Jumprope

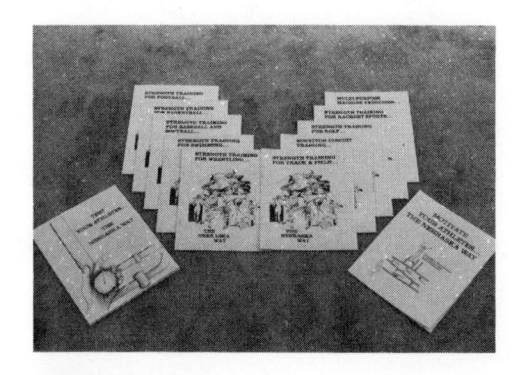

Figure 4.24
Specific Programs from Boyd Epley

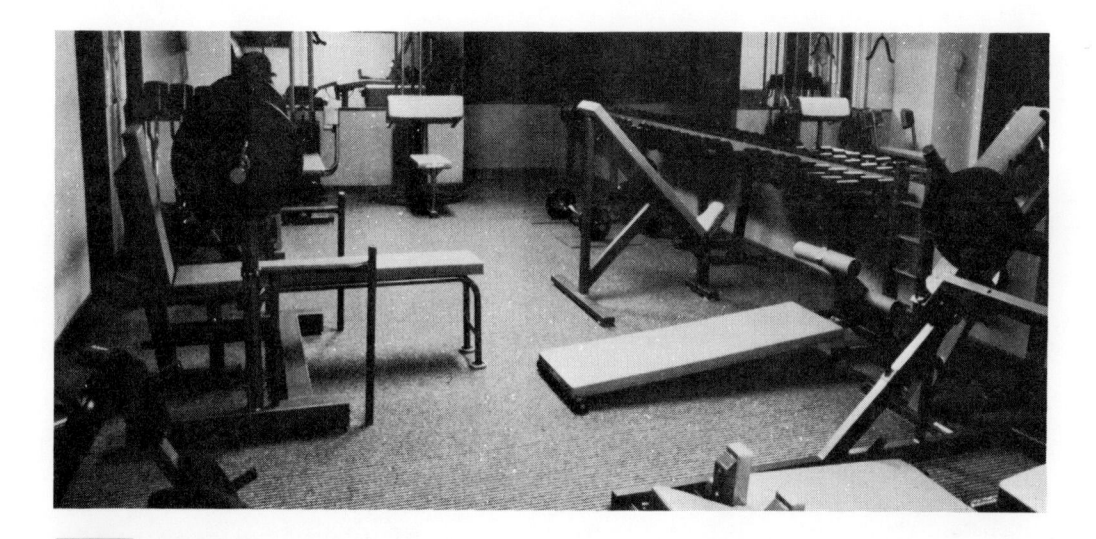

Figure 4.25
Home Exercise Equipment

Home exercise equipment doesn't need to be a rusty old barbell set left out in the garage. Many families are now including beautiful exercise rooms in the design of their homes. There are many types of equipment available within various price ranges. Some are geared more for general fitness; some more for strength. The equipment presented in this chapter is specifically for the development of strength.

Selecting Your Equipment 39

CHAPTER FIVE

Off-Season and In-Season Training

The name of the lifting program you are about to learn is *Split Routine Six-Week Cycle*. Strength training can give you increases in strength and power, as well as muscular endurance, if you train properly. These are all very important aspects in athletics, because if you are able to achieve increases in these areas at an early age, you could be very much ahead of other athletes. As you become bigger, stronger, and faster as a result of your consistent workouts, your confidence in yourself will grow. A split routine six week cycle is the best program you can follow.

Off-Season Training: The Split Routine

The suggested number of workout periods for weight training is normally three per week. Not three successive days, but three alternate ones. For example, a Monday-Wednesday-Friday schedule, or Tuesday-Thursday-Saturday program gives the muscles an opportunity to rest on the off days.

In strength training we use what is called a *split routine*. This is a very efficient and widely-used principle in stimulating gains in strength. It simply means that your program is split so that you work only half your body parts on one day and the other half on the next day. Dividing body parts and working them on separate days allows shorter workouts, as opposed to long, drawn-out workouts that work all body parts in one day. This allows you to include other types of athletic workouts, such as running and speed drills, without overtraining in any one component. The split routine allows half of your body parts to recover and rebuild while you work on the other half of your program.

Following is an example of the recommended split routine.

Monday	*Tuesday*	*Thursday*	*Friday*
Chest	Back	Chest	Back
Legs	Shoulders	Legs	Shoulders
Stomach	Arms	Stomach	Arms

Each week you work out four days, working each body part twice, and allowing at least two days rest for recovery between working a particular muscle. Beginners are usually full of enthusiasm. They sometimes think that, since the four-day split routine works so well, then six days a week must be better. Unfortunately, things don't work that way. Take Wednesday off from lifting, in addition to the weekend, because your body will need the time to build stronger muscles.

Overtraining

One of the biggest deterrents in a strength program is overtraining. If you are constantly working at full intensity, you aren't allowing your body to recover and rebuild. If you train every single day, you might easily overwork a muscle to the point where you would tire it out and tear it down—thus actually reducing its size and strength, rather than building it. Your body's growth process depends upon proper nutrition, sufficient exercise, and adequate rest. If you overdo or neglect any of these aspects, you may not make the progress you desire. Overtraining is common in championship and "weekend" athletes alike. If you have the feeling that you have reached a training plateau where you just aren't making good progress, a change is needed. If you don't feel like training, don't; a setback caused by a poor attitude might be worse for you than taking a day or two off from training. You can lose confidence in yourself, which seriously hampers your progress. To get back on track you'll need to maintain a positive attitude, and setting and achieving realistic goals will help. If you don't reach your goals, don't become too discouraged; adjust them so they are attainable.

Cycling

Cycling is a good way to avoid training plateaus. The theory behind cycling is that by working at a certain intensity, then changing to a different intensity, you create a new overload to your body, which responds with renewed excitability. This switch from one intensity to another is repeated until you have gone through all of the weeks of the training cycle. The cycle is completed in six weeks; then repeated again. Of course, you will be using more weight to start your second cycle than you were at the start of your first training cycle.

Week 1	Week 2	Week 3	Week 4	Week 5	Week 6
10	12	15	15	15	15
			10	12	15

Figure 5.1
Recommended Six-Week Cycle for Beginners

Recommended Six-Week Split Routine Cycle for Beginners

Week One (One Set of 10)

The proper amount of weight to use for each exercise varies with each individual person. Don't be concerned with how much poundage your friends might be using on a particular exercise. You will add heavier weight as you grow stronger, but you are wise in starting with light poundages and gradually increasing each week as you progress through your cycle. First, do a light warm-up set of 6 to 8 repetitions with an extremely light poundage. Then do your set with a poundage you think you can handle for 10 repetitions. At first the exercise movement will seem awkward; you have to allow a bit of time for learning to take effect. Remember to do the exercise properly, with a full range of motion. If you cannot do 10 repetitions without cheating or straining, the weight is too heavy. The correct amount of weight will make you feel that you have done some work, especially on the last few repetitions.

Week Two (One Set of 12)

You've worked each body part twice in Week One, so you should have learned how to perform the exercises properly. You're now ready for a little overload to your muscles. By raising the number of repetitions to 12, your muscles will be forced to do more work. You can probably use the same poundage for each exercise that you used in week one.

Week Three (One Set of 15)

By changing the training load to 15 repetitions, you have again overloaded your muscles. They will be forced to lift the weight more times than in Week Two. You may experience a burning sensation in your muscles on your last few repetitions. This feeling is lactic acid building up in the muscle, and is a sign that you are building endurance in the muscle.

Week Four (Two Sets 15/10)

In addition to your set of 15 repetitions, your program now calls for an additional set of 10 repetitions on each exercise. This additional set is an overload to your muscles, and will cause your muscles to grow stronger. Do both sets for each exercise before you move on to the next exercise, and allow one to two minutes rest between sets and between exercises.

Week Five (Two Sets, 15/12)

Once again the training load is increased, causing your muscles to work harder than they did the previous week. By progressively making the program more difficult in this way, you will experience gains in strength and endurance, even if you use the same poundage for an exercise throughout the entire cycle.

You should be trying to increase the poundage you are using on each exercise as often as you can, however, as long as you are able to perform the recommended number of repetitions.

Week Six (Two Sets 15/15)

You have made your program more difficult each and every week. However, you cannot continue making your program more intense, because you will surely experience a training plateau where you are no longer able to make any progress. You also run a risk of getting mentally and physically burned-out as your program gets harder and harder. Plan to start your cycle over again next week with one set of 10, but increase the poundage you've been using.

Muscle Soreness

It is not uncommon to experience some stiffness and muscle soreness, particularly after your first few workouts. Even advanced lifters oftentimes experience some muscle soreness after a very strenuous workout. This is a good sign because it means you have activated muscle fibers that were not used much before. Don't be surprised if your muscle soreness is greater on the second day after exercising than it is the day immediately following your workout.

Record Your Progress

It is a good idea to keep a regular written record of your workouts to help you monitor your progress. This will also help you know if you are reaching your goals, and allow you to determine how much weight to use on your next workout. A progress chart is provided in figure 5.2 for you to record your workouts.

Exercise Performance Chart for the Beginner

Monday/Thursday Exercises	Mon. Reps	Mon. Wt.Rep	Thur. Wt.Rep	Thur. Reps	Mon. Wt.Rep	Mon. Reps	Thur. Wt.Rep	Thur. Reps	Mon. Wt.Rep	Mon. Reps	Thur. Wt.Rep	Thur. Reps	Mon. Wt.Rep	Mon. Reps	Thur. Wt.Rep
Bench Press	WU			WU		WU		WU		WU		WU		WU	
	10			12		15		10		15		12		15	
Incline Press	WU			WU		WU		WU		WU		WU		WU	
	10			12		15		10		15		12		15	
Squat, Hip Sled or Lunge	WU			WU		WU		WU		WU		WU		WU	
	10			12		15		10		15		12		15	
Leg Extension	WU			WU		WU		WU		WU		WU		WU	
	10			12		15		10		15		12		15	
Leg Curl	WU			WU		WU		WU		WU		WU		WU	
	10			12		15		10		15		12		15	
Sit-Up															

Tuesday/Friday	Reps	Tues.	Fri.	Reps	Tues.	Fri.	Reps	Tues.	Fri.	Reps	Tues.	Fri.	Reps	Tues.	Fri.	Reps	Tues.	Fri.
Exercises		Wt.Rep	Wt.Rep		Wt.Rep	Wt.Rep		Wt.Rep	Wt.Rep		Wt.Rep	Wt.Rep		Wt.Rep	Wt.Rep		Wt.Rep	Wt.Rep
	WU			WU			WU			WU			WU			WU		
Upright Row	10			12			15			15			15			15		
										10			12			15		
	WU			WU			WU			WU			WU			WU		
Military Press	10			12			15			15			15			15		
										10			12			15		
	WU			WU			WU			WU			WU			WU		
Lateral Raise	10			12			15			15			15			15		
										10			12			15		
	WU			WU			WU			WU			WU			WU		
Bent-Over Raise	10			12			15			15			15			15		
										10			12			15		
	WU			WU			WU			WU			WU			WU		
Curl	10			12			15			15			15			15		
										10			12			15		
	WU			WU			WU			WU			WU			WU		
Tricep Extension	10			12			15			15			15			15		
										10			12			15		

Figure 5.2
Exercise Performance Chart. Do a light warm-up set before each new exercise, and record the weight in the WU column.

Advanced Exercise Performance Chart

Monday/Thursday Exercises	Reps	Mon. Wt.Rep	Thur. Wt.Rep	Reps	Mon. Wt.Rep	Thur. Wt.Rep	Reps	Mon. Wt.Rep	Thur. Wt.Rep	Reps	Mon. Wt.Rep	Thur. Wt.Rep	Reps	Mon. Wt.Rep	Thur. Wt.Rep
Bench Press	15			15			12								
				12			10								
							8								
Incline Press	15			15			12								
				12			10								
							8								
Squat, Hip Sled or Lunge	15			15			12								
				12			10								
							8								
Leg Extension	15			15			12								
				12			10								
							8								
Leg Curl	15			15			12								
				12			10								
							8								
Sit-Up															

Tuesday/Friday Exercises	Reps	Tues. Wt.Rep	Fri. Wt.Rep	Reps	Tues. Wt.Rep	Fri. Wt.Rep	Reps	Tues. Wt.Rep	Fri. Wt.Rep	Reps	Tues. Wt.Rep	Fri. Wt.Rep
Upright Row	15			15			12					
				12			10					
Military Press	15			15			12					
				12			10					
Lateral Raise	15			15			12					
				12			10					
Bent-Over Raise	15			15			12					
				12			10					
Curl	15			15			12					
				12			10					
Tricep Extension	15			15			12					
				12			10					

Figure 5.3
Advanced Exercise Performance Chart. Do a light warm-up set before each new exercise.

Off-Season and In-Season Training   47

Who Is the Strongest?

It is human nature to want to see how much weight you can lift. Unfortunately, when young athletes get together to train there is frequently a contest to find out who is the strongest. It is not wise for a young person to start lifting the heaviest weight he can handle right away; and it is not necessary for you to see how much you can lift for one repetition. In fact, that is the fastest way for you to receive an injury. You only have one body, so treat it with respect, and follow your cycling program as outlined. The beginner's cycle starts with one set for each exercise, and progresses according to the training cycle, adding another set to each exercise. After you've been through the beginning cycle a few times you may want to increase your number of sets to three. This, of course, is not advised for the beginner, but rather for the more advanced trainee who has had more experience. It is very important to note here that heavy resistance should not be used by young athletes whose long bones are still growing. A traumatic injury to the epiphyseal disc at this time can lead to stunted limb growth, and a permanent handicap. The younger the athlete, the greater the emphasis should be on lighter weights and higher repetitions.

Puberty, and the resulting growth spurt, begins in girls between ten and twelve years of age, and about one to two years later than this in boys. Since this is the time when the limbs are growing the fastest, any strength training done at this time should be done with great care. The activity of the epiphyseal discs slows greatly during new bone formation following the growth spurt, and eventually they stop producing bone altogether. Disc closure occurs in females at about eighteen years of age; in males at about twenty years. Maximum poundages can be used after pubescent growth is complete. This indicates that females can start using heavy poundages at a younger age than males, since their skeletal development period begins and ends sooner. Young athletes should concentrate on their recommended cycles, and be sure to lift the weight using proper form.

In-Season Training: Strength Maintenance

An in-season program is a little different from the six-week split routine cycle used in the off-season. Your main goal in-season is to *maintain* your strength throughout the season. The two major changes for your in-season program involve 1.) not using a split routine and 2.) not doing a cycle. Do all of your exercises twice a week during the season. For example, if your competition is on Friday, your lifting days should be Monday and Wednesday. Rather than trying to cycle through different levels of intensity each week, simply do one or two sets of 10 to 12 repetitions on each exercise. This strength maintenance program requires far less time than the strength development cycle, which will give you more time to develop your specific sport skills.

A common mistake some athletes make is to stop strength training after they enter their competitive season, thinking that they will retain their strength. Unless you are consistent with your strength training, strength is lost at the same rate as it is gained. However, if strength is built over a long period of time, it becomes firmly secured and tends to be lost very slowly. Generally speaking, a good strength maintenance program can maintain 90 to 95 percent of the strength gained during the off-season.

Approximately ninety-six hours after your final workout, your strength level will begin to fall off. Although a strength loss of 3 to 5 percent a week does not seem like much over the course of an entire athletic season, these small losses add up to a very large loss in strength. Because of this, you should think in terms of a year-round strength training program.

CHAPTER SIX

What to Do Your First Day

I realize you are anxious to start right away on your split routine six-week cycle program, but there are a few things you should do before you actually start your cycle.

Since your cycle starts on a Monday, it would be a good idea to get your family together on Sunday to get organized so you'll be ready to go the next day. I'd like you to do several things:

1. Take your measurements.
2. Learn the stretching routine.
3. Practice the lifting exercises with a bar only.

Measurements

Take your measurements every six weeks, at the start of each new cycle, to monitor any physical changes. You may have to ask someone else to help you, since it is difficult to ensure that the tape is not crooked. Measurements should be taken before you do any exercise, not after. The tape should be laid on the skin and pulled snug, but not too tight. Your body weight should be taken in the nude, or in underwear if necessary. Your chest measurement should be taken at the largest part, with the tape just above the nipples in front and straight across the back. Breathe normally and do not flex the back muscles during this measurement. Your stomach measurement should be taken at the smallest part while you are standing. Do not suck in your stomach during the measurement. Your hips should be measured around the fullest part of the buttocks while standing. Your arm should be raised to shoulder level, with the bicep fully contracted, the fist clenched and turned down. The measurement should be taken so the tape is straight up and down at the point measuring the greatest size of the bicep. Your thigh muscle should be relaxed. Your calf measurement should be taken at the largest part, with the foot flat on the floor. Write down your measurements each time on the chart that is provided in table 6.1 and be sure to record the date.

Table 6.1
Progress Records

Progress Record of _____

Age	_____	Age	_____	Age	_____
Date	_____	Date	_____	Date	_____
Body weight	_____	Body weight	_____	Body weight	_____
Chest	_____	Chest	_____	Chest	_____
Stomach	_____	Stomach	_____	Stomach	_____
Hips	_____	Hips	_____	Hips	_____
Right arm	_____	Right arm	_____	Right arm	_____
Left arm	_____	Left arm	_____	Left arm	_____
Right thigh	_____	Right thigh	_____	Right thigh	_____
Left thigh	_____	Left thigh	_____	Left thigh	_____
Right calf	_____	Right calf	_____	Right calf	_____
Left calf	_____	Left calf	_____	Left calf	_____

Table 6.1—*Continued*

Progress Record of _____

Age _____	Age _____	Age _____
Date _____	Date _____	Date _____
Body weight _____	Body weight _____	Body weight _____
Chest _____	Chest _____	Chest _____
Stomach _____	Stomach _____	Stomach _____
Hips _____	Hips _____	Hips _____
Right arm _____	Right arm _____	Right arm _____
Left arm _____	Left arm _____	Left arm _____
Right thigh _____	Right thigh _____	Right thigh _____
Left thigh _____	Left thigh _____	Left thigh _____
Right calf _____	Right calf _____	Right calf _____
Left calf _____	Left calf _____	Left calf _____

Stretching Routine

After you've gotten all your measurements out of the way, it is time to learn the stretching routine that you'll want to do at the beginning of each workout.

The recommended stretching routine actually serves a dual purpose. First, the stretching exercises prepare your body for your exercise program by raising both the body and deep muscle temperatures. Secondly, the routine helps you increase your current flexibility, which could help you improve your athletic performance. This stretching routine should be done before each training session.

Note: Even though this stretching routine will warm up the body and prepare it for general exercise, you will still want to do a light warm-up set on each lifting exercise you're going to do. You can't warm-up the chest muscle by doing a set of squats. A warm-up set is something you need to make a regular part of your lifting program. The beginning progress chart in chapter 5 provides a space for you to record your warm-up set. This will serve as a reminder for you. The advanced progress chart provided in chapter 5 does not include a space to record a warm-up set because the advanced athlete does the warm-up set automatically and doesn't need a reminder.

I've stated that following the stretching routine will improve your flexibility, but why is more flexibility important to you? Let's ask an expert on flexible athletes. Francis Allen is the head gymnastics coach for the University of Nebraska. His teams have won five straight national championships in gymnastics; two of his gymnasts won gold medals in the 1984 Olympics.

Francis says:

> The need to improve flexibility in children is many times overlooked. Flexibility is very important at any age. Children have longitudinal bone growth and as the bones grow the muscular tendinous unit remains tight. Almost all children will experience tightness in either the back, heel cords or hamstrings. A good stretching program should be done daily to improve flexibility in these areas.

How can an improvement in your flexibility help you become a better athlete?

1. Improvement of performance. An increase of flexibility in your hamstring and shoulder area will increase your range of motion, permitting greater potential for speed improvement. This will be important to you when performing the drills that increase your running speed (chapter 9).

2. Prevention of injuries. There are many situations in sport activities where a muscle is forced to stretch beyond its normal active limits. If the muscle does not have enough elasticity to compensate, an injury might occur.

3. Development of greater strength. The development of strength throughout the full range of motion requires flexibility of the joints involved. Actually, proper strength training, when combined with your stretching routine, will also help improve your flexibility.

4. Development of better coordination. In chapter 2 you saw that muscles work in pairs. Poor coordination may be due to a low rate of flexibility development, resulting in a lack of coordination between the contraction and relaxation of the muscles (agonist versus antagonist).

When you do your stretching routine, you must stretch within your limits without straining. Stretching is not a contest, it is entirely individual. There are three categories in stretching: 1.) the easy stretch 2.) the developmental stretch, and 3.) the drastic stretch. Begin each position with the easy stretch. You should be totally relaxed without any discomfort. Gradually move into the developmental stretch, where you will feel the stretch become more intense without causing actual pain. Do not use the drastic stretch; the body would be uneasy, it would be impossible to relax, and an injury may result.

There is a difference between the feeling of a stretch and pain. When you stretch, it should be to a point where you feel an easy stretch—then hold and relax by thinking about the feeling of the stretch. As the feeling of the stretch changes to a milder stretch, you should stretch a little farther. If you go too far it will hurt, and you will not be able to relax. You cannot relax if you are straining or in pain.

Four-Minute Stretching Routine

Elbow Behind Head

Procedure Pull your elbow behind your head and hold for an easy stretch of ten seconds with one arm, then switch arms.

Value The primary muscle stretched is the tricep, as illustrated in figure 6.1 by the little dots.

Total Time Twenty seconds.

Side Stretch

Procedure With both hands extended overhead, slowly bend at the waist as you gently pull your top hand toward the floor. Stretch each side ten seconds.

Value The primary muscles stretched are the lateral muscles of the abdominal wall.

Total Time Twenty seconds.

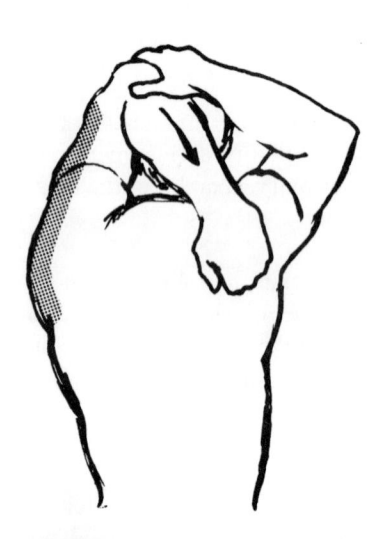

Figure 6.1
Elbow Behind Head

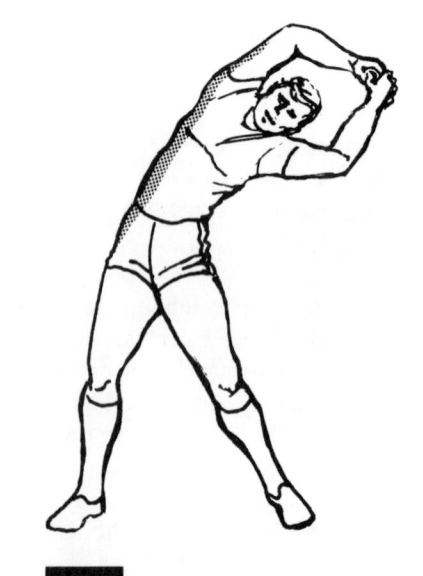

Figure 6.2
Side Stretch

Toe Touch

Procedure From a standing position with the legs straight or slightly bent, slowly bend at the waist until you feel an easy stretch in the back of your legs. Don't go down too fast, or so far that you feel pain. Do not bounce in an attempt to go farther down.

Value The primary muscle stretched is the hamstring.

Total Time Thirty seconds.

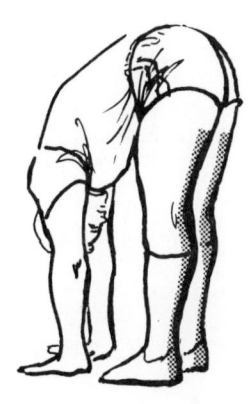

Figure 6.3
Toe Touch

Seated Toe Touch

Procedure Sit down with your heels four to eight inches apart. Keep your legs straight as you bend forward at the waist. Try to touch your ankles. Once you can, then try to reach your toes, then your heels.

Value The primary muscle stretched is the hamstring.

Total time Twenty seconds.

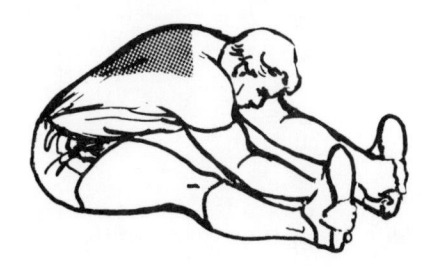

Figure 6.4
Seated Toe Touch

Spinal Twist

Procedure From a seated position, place one foot across the opposite knee so that it is flat on the ground. Then brace the opposite arm against the bent leg and twist away as you apply pressure to the bent leg with the back of your arm. Hold for ten seconds, then switch legs.

Value The primary area being stretched is the lower back.

Total time Twenty seconds.

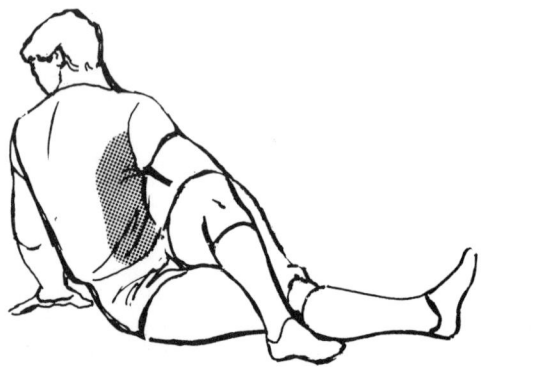

Figure 6.5
Spinal Twist

Hurdle Forward

Procedure Bend one leg so the heel is in the crotch area. Then lean forward at the waist, keeping the other leg straight. Attempt to reach your ankle or foot, pulling your chin down toward the knee of the straight leg. Hold for ten seconds and switch.

Value This position allows you to bring a great degree of stretch to the hamstring and lower back.

Total time Twenty seconds.

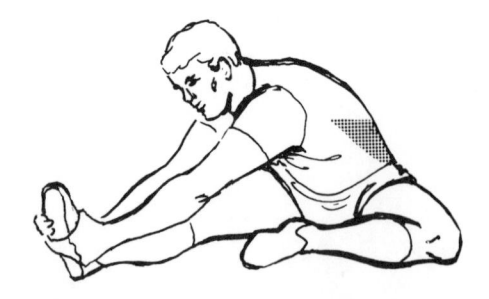

Figure 6.6
Hurdle Forward

Cross-Over

Procedure Use your right hand on the outside of the left thigh to gently pull the leg down. Be sure to keep your left shoulder flat on the ground. Hold for ten seconds and switch legs.

Value The primary muscles stretched are the lower back erectors.

Total time Twenty seconds.

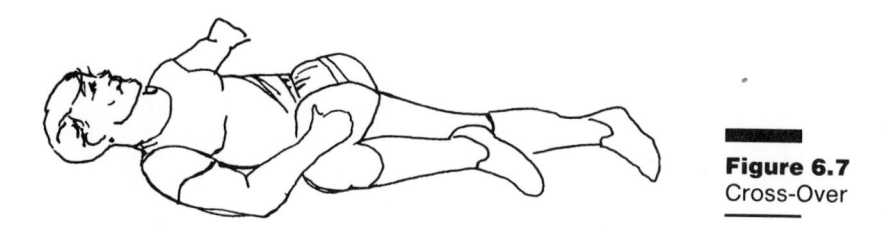

Figure 6.7 Cross-Over

Leg Spread

Procedure Sit up with your legs straight out and split your legs as far out as possible. Keep your feet upright and relaxed. Then slowly lean forward until you feel a stretch on the insides of your legs. Hold for twenty seconds. Sit up straight again, then reach out to your right foot with your legs still as far apart as possible. Hold to the right for fifteen seconds. Sit up straight again, then reach to your left foot and hold for fifteen seconds.

Value The primary muscle being stretched is the hamstring.

Total time Fifty seconds.

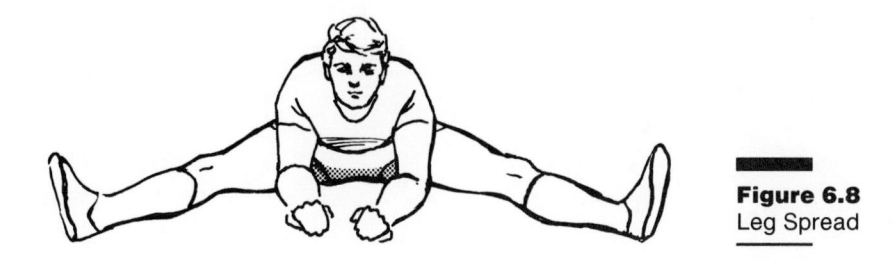

Figure 6.8 Leg Spread

Squat

Procedure Squat down as far as you can, keeping your heels flat on the ground. First try to touch your buttocks to the ground, then try to touch your elbows to the ground. Hold for twenty seconds.

Value The primary area being stretched is the hip area.

Total time Twenty seconds.

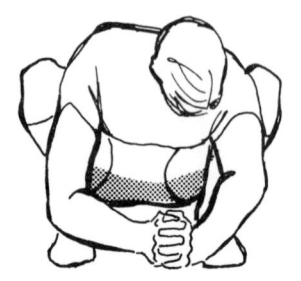

Figure 6.9
Squat

One Foot Forward

Procedure Position yourself with one leg forward with a bent knee. Your knee should be directly over the ankle. Your foot should be flat on the ground; your other leg directly behind you with the knee touching the ground. Now move your hips slowly forward and hold for ten seconds, then switch legs.

Value The primary muscles being stretched are the quadricep and hamstring, but this is also good for your ankle.

Total time Twenty seconds.

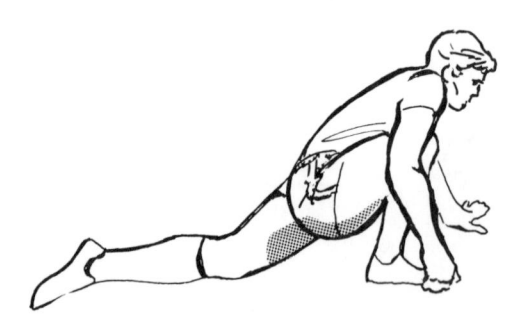

Figure 6.10
One Foot Forward

Lifting Exercises with a Bar Only

Before you officially start your cycling program, I'd like you to practice all your exercises with a bar only. By using an extremely light poundage you'll get the feel of the proper form without straining. Concentrate on making a complete extension and contraction of each muscle as you perform each exercise. This good form that you are establishing is the same that you will use when you exercise with more poundage after you officially start your cycle on Monday, and it is the same form that you'll use years from now. Bouncing the bar off the chest, or arching the back, are common "cheating" techniques. By incorporating these kinds of cheating techniques, the muscle does not do the actual work, and does not receive the full benefit of the exercise. Such a practice is very unwise because of the possibility of joint and muscle injury. Always use good lifting form on all your exercises. Take time to practice your form on the recommended exercises that are listed in chapters 7 and 8.

CHAPTER SEVEN

Monday-Thursday Lifting Exercises

This chapter includes the six exercises that are the most important for chest, leg, and stomach development. These six exercises are to be performed on Monday and again on Thursday of each week in your off-season program.

1. Bench press
2. Incline press
3. Squat, hip sled, or lunge
4. Leg extension
5. Leg curl
6. Sit-up

Over the years I have had the opportunity to work with some outstanding athletes. I have asked a few of them to comment on the nature of the exercises that I am recommending for your lifting program. In addition to their comments on each of the six major exercises, I have provided several supplementary exercises for your consideration.

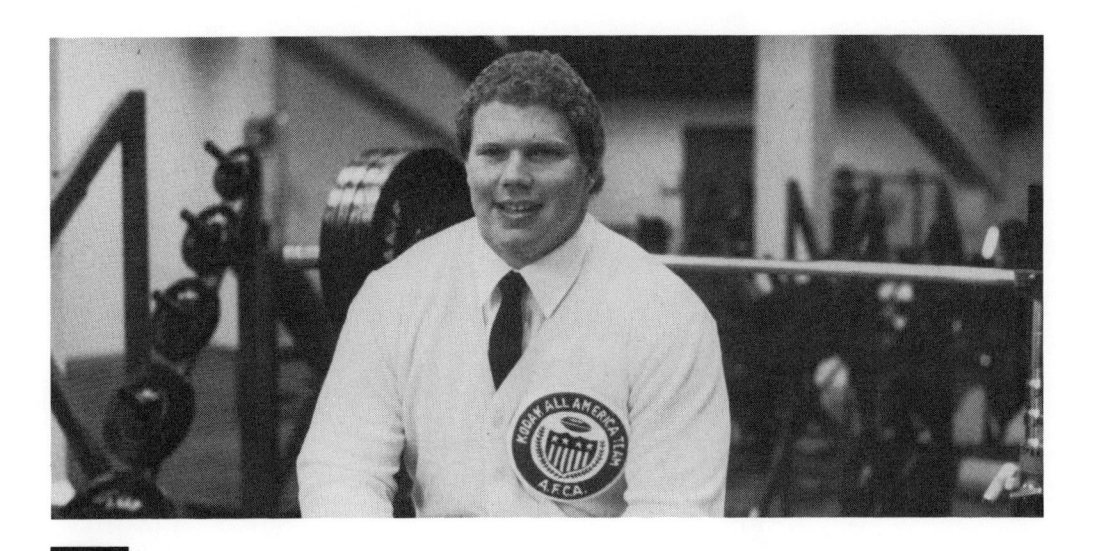

Figure 7.1
Dave Rimington was the first player to win the Outland Award twice.

Recommended Exercises for the Chest

Bench Press (7:1)

The bench press is the most widely recognized exercise for chest development. If someone were asked "How strong are you?", he would most likely reply by saying how much weight he could bench press.

Dave Rimington, center for the Cincinnati Bengals, was one of the strongest athletes I ever worked with at the University of Nebraska. Dave, who had the benefit of a good high school strength program, bench pressed 340 pounds while he was still in high school. Four years later he set a Big Eight centers record on the bench press by lifting 435 pounds. Dave Rimington says, "Young athletes should take the time to learn good technique before attempting heavy poundages. Don't bounce the bar off your chest, or raise your buttocks off the bench. Let your pectoral muscles do the work." Dave Rimington set a standard I am not sure anyone will ever match. He is the only athlete to ever win the Outland Trophy (emblematic of the nation's outstanding lineman) twice. Dave added the Lombardi Award to his list of honors his senior year in college, in addition to being named to the Academic All-American and All-American Strength Teams. Dave weighed only 220 pounds coming out of high school, but was a muscular 300 pounds at the 1983 Orange Bowl during his senior year in college. Dave set a tremendous example in the weight room, on the field, and in the classroom. Dave says, "Young athletes should concentrate on the basic program as outlined in this book. As you gain in maturity and experience, you can customize your workouts to suit you better."

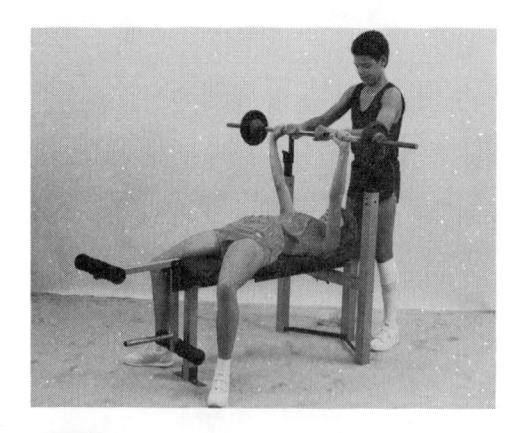

Figure 7.2
Bench Press—Start

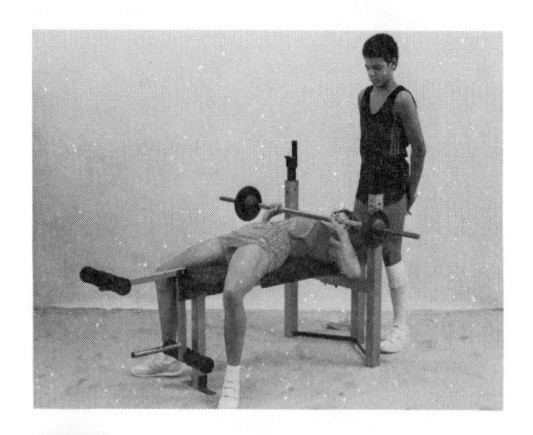

Figure 7.3
Bench Press—Chest Position

Procedure Obtain a grip wider than your shoulders but not wider than the rings on the bar (if you have an Olympic bar). While lying on your back on the bench, position yourself toward the end of the bench. Reach back and grasp the bar; leave the head and buttocks on the bench. Pull the shoulder blades inward as you push the chest upward. Place the shoulder blades on the bench; place the feet out wide. Your eyes should be looking up at the near edge of the bar. Try to get a high arch in the back as the buttocks are set on the bench. You are now ready to lift. When lowering the bar to the chest, allow the bar to lightly "touch" on the lower chest area. Keep the elbows pointed outward. After touching the chest, extend the bar to full arm's length. When looking at the bar from the side, there should be a slight curve backwards in the pattern of motion of the bar from the lower part of the chest to almost over the eyes at full extension of the arms.

Value Major development from this exercise will be to the pectoral muscles (chest), with some development to the anterior deltoid (front of shoulder) and triceps (back of arm). This is a major exercise in your program.

Equipment Although an Olympic bar should be used for best results, a regular bar is fine for the home gym. Bench press benches vary a great deal in quality and cost. Be sure to obtain one that is sturdy enough to handle the heavy poundages you will use as you get older and stronger, in addition to your increased body weight.

Safety A spotter must be used for this exercise—either one spotter positioned as shown, or two spotters, one on each end of the bar. You would be wise to use dumbbells rather than a barbell if lifting alone. Most benches found in the home are of a narrow stance as shown. Most colleges use a wider stance bench, which is known as a competition bench. When using a narrow bench, you must be careful not to unload one side of the bar before unloading the other, or the bar could flip off of the bench.

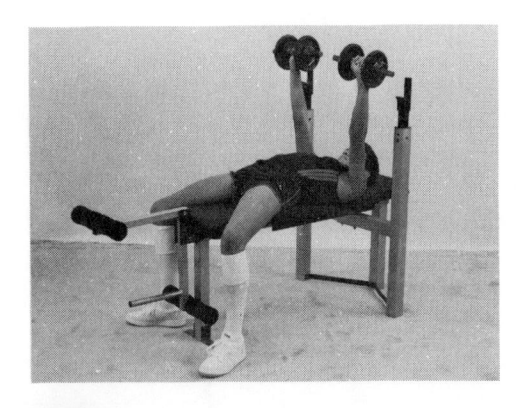

Figure 7.4
Dumbbell Press—Start

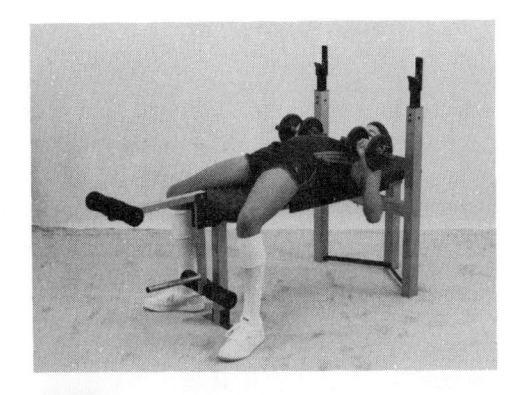

Figure 7.5
Dumbbell Press—Chest Position

Supplementary Exercises for the Bench Press

In addition to this major exercise, here are several supplementary exercises for you that work the same muscle group. I would prefer that you do the major exercises in your program; however, I want you to be aware of the supplementary ones, also.

      7:1A Dumbbell bench press

      7:1B Lying lateral raise

      7:1C Close grip bench press

Dumbbell Bench Press (7:1A)

Procedure While lying on the bench, position yourself toward the end of the bench, leaving your head and buttocks on the bench. Place the shoulder blades on the bench with the feet shoulder-width apart. The eyes should be looking up at the dumbbells. Try to get a high arch in the back as the buttocks are set on the bench. Start with the dumbbells at full arms length just above the chest. Lower the dumbbells to the chest, allowing them to lightly "touch" on the lower chest area. Keep the elbows pointed outward as the dumbbells are extended to full arm's length. When looking at the dumbbells from the side, there should be a slight curve backwards in the pattern of the motion of these dumbbells as they are extended up.

Value Development from this exercise will be to the pectoral muscles (chest), with some development to the anterior deltoid (front of shoulder) and triceps (back of arm). This is a supplementary chest exercise, and a substitute for the bench press with a barbell if you are lifting alone.

Equipment A pair of dumbbells and a bench press bench are needed for this exercise.

Lying Lateral Raise (7:1B)

Procedure Lie on your back and hold the dumbbells at arm's length with the palms facing each other. The elbows should be slightly bent. Lower the dumbbells out to the side until they are about four inches lower than the chest. From this position pull the dumbbells upward and together while maintaining just a slight bend in the elbow. This exercise should be done slowly and smoothly.

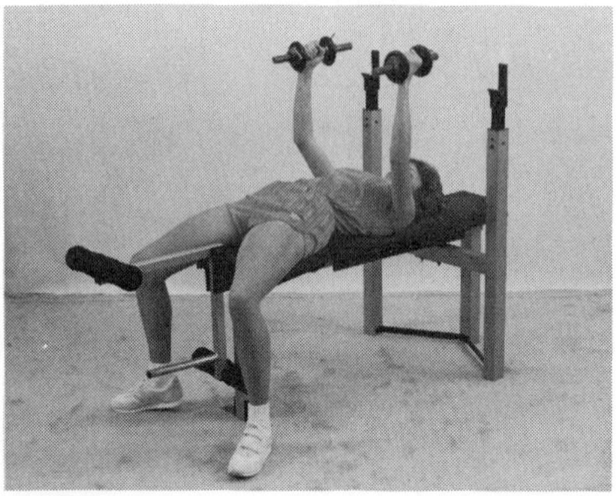

Figure 7.6
Lying Lateral Raise—Start

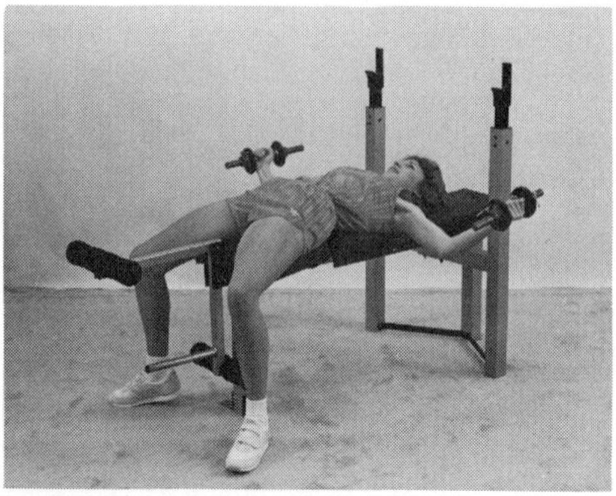

Figure 7.7
Lying Lateral Raise—Chest Position

Value This exercise will develop the outer fibers of the pectoralis major muscle (outer chest). This is a supplementary chest exercise.

Equipment A pair of dumbbells and a bench are required for this exercise.

Safety A slight bend in the elbow will cause less stress to be put on the elbow joint; there should not be any hyperextension of the elbows.

Close Grip Bench Press (7:1C)

Procedure The close grip bench press is very similar to the regular bench press. The hand spacing is closer (four to six inches apart), for the close grip. As the bar is lowered to the chest, the upper arms and elbows are held close to the upper body until the bar touches the chest. This exercise should be done slowly and smoothly.

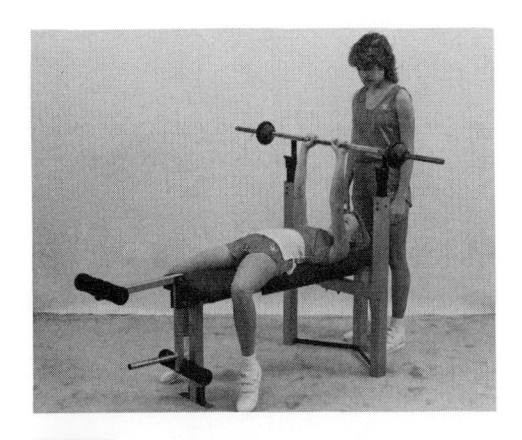

Figure 7.8
Close Grip Bench Press—
Start

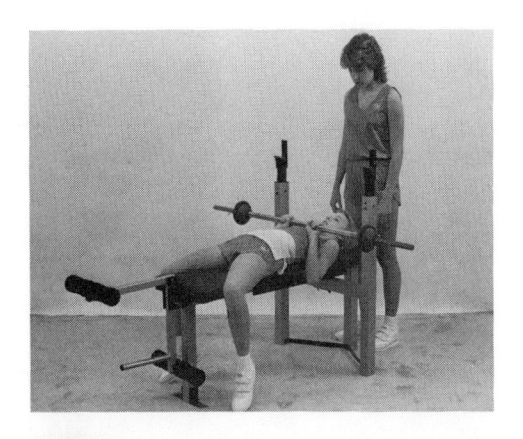

Figure 7.9
Close Grip Bench Press—
Chest Position

Value This exercise will develop the inner fibers of the chest, and will affect the outer head of the tricep. This is a supplementary chest exercise.

Equipment A barbell is needed for the close grip bench press. A wide stance bench would be more favorable than a narrow stance bench for this exercise because the narrow standards are right where you want your hands to be. It is possible to have spotters hand you the barbell when using a narrow stance bench.

Safety Be careful not to pinch your hands when returning the bar to the standards. A spotter should be used for this exercise.

Incline Press (7:2)

The incline press is much like the bench press, however it will concentrate more on the upper fibers of your chest. I recommmend you use a 45 degree angle for the incline press, which makes this exercise the midpoint between a shoulder press and a bench press. An incline setting of less than 45 degrees will work more on the chest, while a more vertical setting will bring in the shoulder mmuscles more, and not work the chest quite as much as you want.

Shot putters and offensive linemen usually rely quite heavily on the incline press to give them the upper chest strength that they need. Dean Steinkuhler says, "The young athlete should get started lifting in junior high school, but he should learn the proper techniques for lifting first." Dean won both the Outland Trophy and the Lombardi Award during his senior year in college. Dean was from a town in Nebraska so small that there wasn't even a high

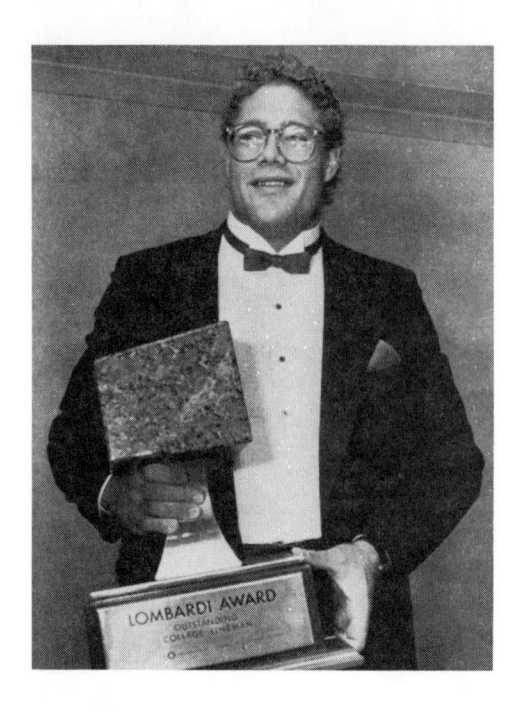

Figure 7.10
Dean Steinkuhler adds the Lombardi Award to his Outland.

school, let alone a strength program. Dean had to travel from Burr to Sterling to go to school, where he played eight-man football. He did not have the benefit of a good strength program in high school like Dave Rimington did. Dean says,

"I never really lifted weights until I came to the university in 1979. Even though I enjoy the bench press and have improved from 225 pounds to 365 pounds, the incline press has probably been more important to me as an offensive lineman, because you push up more than you push out. I needed strength in my chest and arms, and the incline press has done that for me. The first time I did the incline press I could only use 90 pounds."

During his senior year in college, Dean did 340 pounds on the incline press, having increased his body weight from 215 pounds as a freshman to 275 pounds as a senior.

Procedure Use an overhand grip like you do on the bench press, with about the same hand spacing (or in a little closer). Keep the elbows pointed out as the bar is lowered to the upper chest. Then press the bar upward and slightly backward. The bar should pass two to three inches from the chin on both the upward and downward strokes. Watch the bar with the eyes as it is extended to arm's length. This exercise should be performed slowly and smoothly.

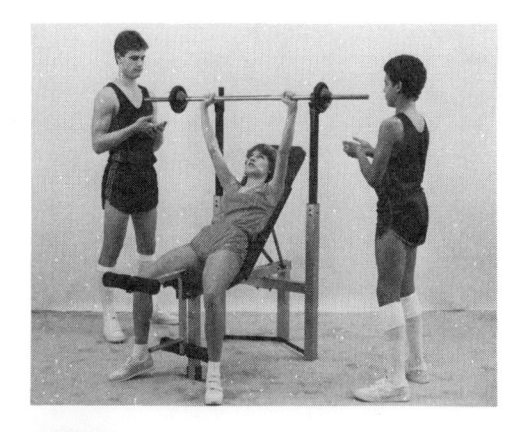

Figure 7.11
Incline Press—Start

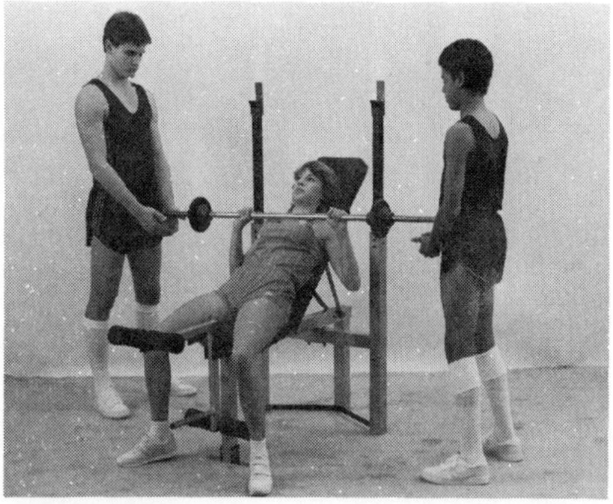

Figure 7.12
Incline Press—Chest Position

Value Major development from this exercise will be to the upper fibers of the pectoral muscle, with some benefit to the anterior deltoid and the tricep. This is a major exercise in your program, and should be done in addition to the bench press.

Equipment An incline bench and barbell are needed for this exercise. The standard incline bench is set at a 45 degree angle. Most benches designed for home use are designed to adjust to a 45 degree incline. Be sure you select a sturdy one that will support not only the weight you are lifting, but also your body weight.

Safety You will need a spotter from behind, or two spotters, one on each end of the bar. You would be wise to use dumbbells rather than a barbell, if lifting alone.

Supplementary Exercises for the Incline Press

      7:2A Dumbbell incline press

      7:2B Incline lateral raise (flys)

Dumbbell Incline Press (7:2A)

Procedure The dumbbells require more balance than the barbell incline press, and require independent coordination of each arm. The dumbbells are held straight up at arm's length, with the palms facing forward. The dumbbells should be six to eight inches apart at the starting position. The dumbbells are then lowered to the shoulder as low as possible with the

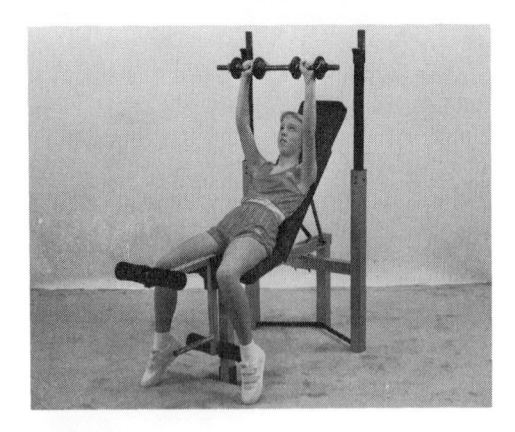

Figure 7.13
Dumbbell Incline Press—
Start

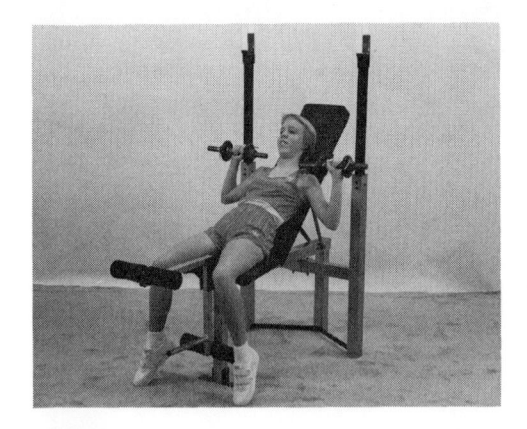

Figure 7.14
Dumbbell Incline Press—
Chest Position

elbows straight out to the side. When the dumbbells are lowered like this, it will put a greater stretch on the chest muscles because the hands are lower than they would be with the barbell. The dumbbells are then pressed slightly backward and upward at the same time.

Value This exercise will develop the upper fibers of the chest. This is a supplementary chest exercise.

Equipment A pair of dumbbells and an incline bench are required for this exercise.

Safety This exercise should be done in place of the incline press if lifting alone.

Incline Lateral Raise (Flys) (7:2B)

Procedure From the incline position, hold the dumbbells at arm's length with the palms facing each other. The elbows should be slightly bent as you lower the dumbbells out to the side until they are about four inches lower than the chest. From this position, pull the dumbbells upward and together, while maintaining just a slight bend in the elbow. This exercise should be done slowly and smoothly.

Value This exercise will develop the outside portion of the upper pectoralis major muscle (the upper portion of the outer chest). This is a supplementary chest exercise.

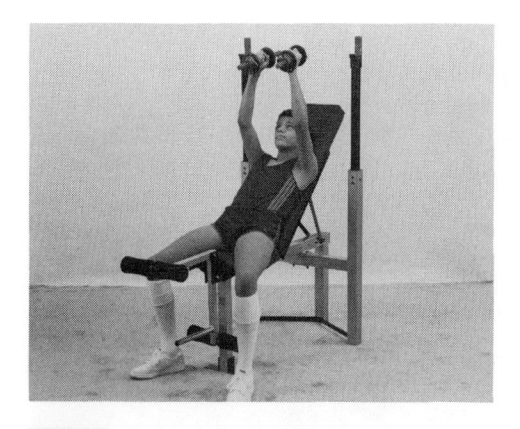

Figure 7.15
Incline Lateral Raise—Start

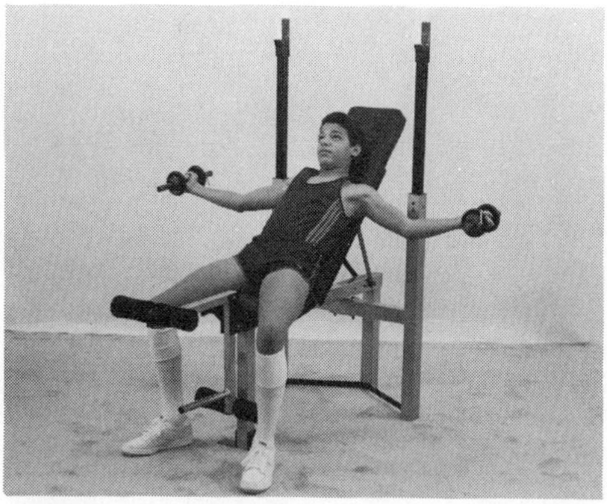

Figure 7.16
Incline Lateral Raise—Chest Position

Equipment A pair of dumbbells and an incline bench are required for this exercise.

Safety A slight bend in the elbow will cause less stress to be put on the elbow joint.

Recommended Exercises for the Legs

Squat, Hip Sled, or Lunge (7:3)

Although I am presenting a choice of three major exercises for your third exercise, the squat is probably the best overall exercise for leg development. Unfortunately, most young athletes do not have a squat rack or squat cage in their homes. This exercise requires two spotters (one on each side of the bar) to help you put the bar back on the uprights when you are finished with your set. Most of the time you won't have two spotters around when you need them at home to spot you on the squat. Therefore, the squat—even though it may be the best exercise for leg development—may not be the best exercise for your situation at home.

When I was first getting started as Strength and Conditioning Coach at Nebraska, an extremely talented freshman named Johnny Rodgers came in. He weighed only 155 pounds and only ran the 40-yard dash in 4.8 seconds, but he was exciting to watch. Freshmen were not eligible for varsity competition back then, which is really unfortunate because the fans only got to watch Johnny run for three years. Johnny set many NCAA records and had a tremendous career, capped by scoring four touchdowns as a 178 pound senior against Notre Dame in the Orange Bowl. He was All-American twice, helped Nebraska win two national

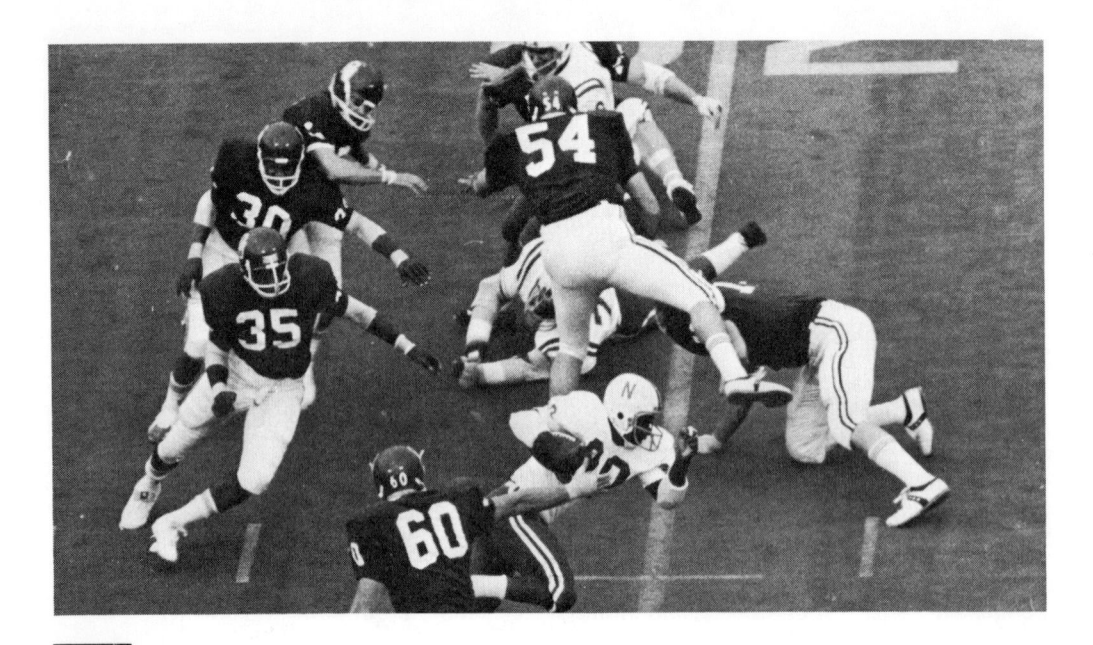

Figure 7.17
Squat. Johnny Rodgers, 1972 Heisman Trophy winner, shows a burst of power.

championships, and was the 1972 Heisman Trophy winner. Johnny was named the outstanding player in the Canadian Football League before finishing up his playing days with the San Diego Chargers. Johnny Rodgers says:

> I came down from a 4.8 "40" to a 4.4 "40" by doing squats. I'm quite sure that doing squats greatly contributed to my athletic abilities. My career in sports was cut short due to knee injuries, but I'm convinced that if I had continued the squat exercises I was doing in Nebraska, it would have lengthened my career and added $700,000 to my income.

Squat

Procedure Position the bar on the back not more than one inch below the top of the shoulders. Remove the bar from the rack by extending the legs and taking slow steps backwards. Position the feet shoulder width apart, or slightly wider, with the toes pointed slightly outward. Keeping the head and elbows up, slowly squat to a position where the middle thigh is parallel to the floor (if using a squat stool, set accordingly). **Note:** If you use a stool, make sure to just touch the stool. Do not bounce. Keep the back as flat as possible by drawing the shoulder blades together. Return to the starting position by keeping an upright posture and extending the legs. Rack the weight slowly.

Figure 7.18
Squat—Start

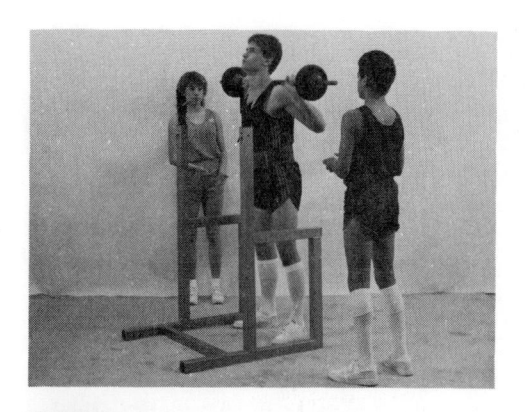

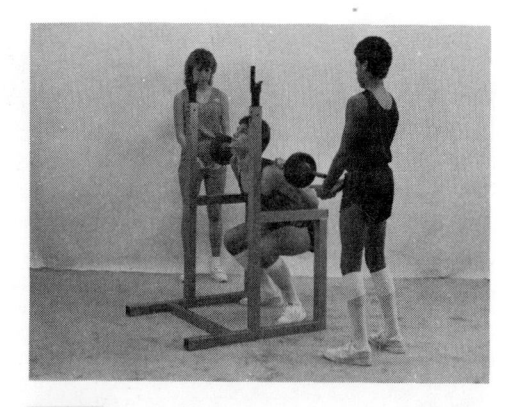

Figure 7.19
Squat—Parallel Position

Value This exercise will develop the quadriceps (thighs), gluteus maximus (hips), and hamstrings (back of leg). This is a major exercise for most programs.

Equipment An Olympic bar (or a standard bar), a squat rack, squat cage, squat uprights, or a power rack are needed for this exercise.

Safety If the exercise is done outside the squat cage or power rack, a minimum of two spotters are required. Three would be ideal: one on either side of the bar, and one directly behind the lifter. If the exercise is done inside a power rack or squat cage, it is still a good idea to have two spotters present. A supportive lumbar lifting belt is recommended for this exercise.

Hip Sled

If you are fortunate enough to have access to a hip sled, you can work your legs much more safely, and no spotters will be necessary. While I recommend the squat as a major exercise for you when done properly with spotters, I do not recommend testing leg strength on the squat. On test day, when our athletes determine their maximum strength for one repetition, we use the hip sled. The hip sled can also be used to develop leg strength. Merlene Ottey, a world class sprinter, says, "Leg strength is very important in athletics. My best is 510 pounds on the hip sled. A typical hip sled workout for me would include 385 pounds for five, 400 pounds for three. I feel this strength has really helped me make a difference in my running." Merlene Ottey has won thirteen individual NCAA titles during her career at Nebraska, and she set three world records during her freshman year alone. She has seven brothers and sisters in her family, but she is the only one that was able to go to college. Her strength training has been extremely important to her. Merlene is a classic example of how strength training has made a great athlete even better. Merlene won a bronze medal in the 200 meters at both the 1980 and 1984 Olympic Games. In addition to its value for testing and for developing leg strength, the hip sled was shown to improve running speed in a 1979 test of Nebraska athletes.

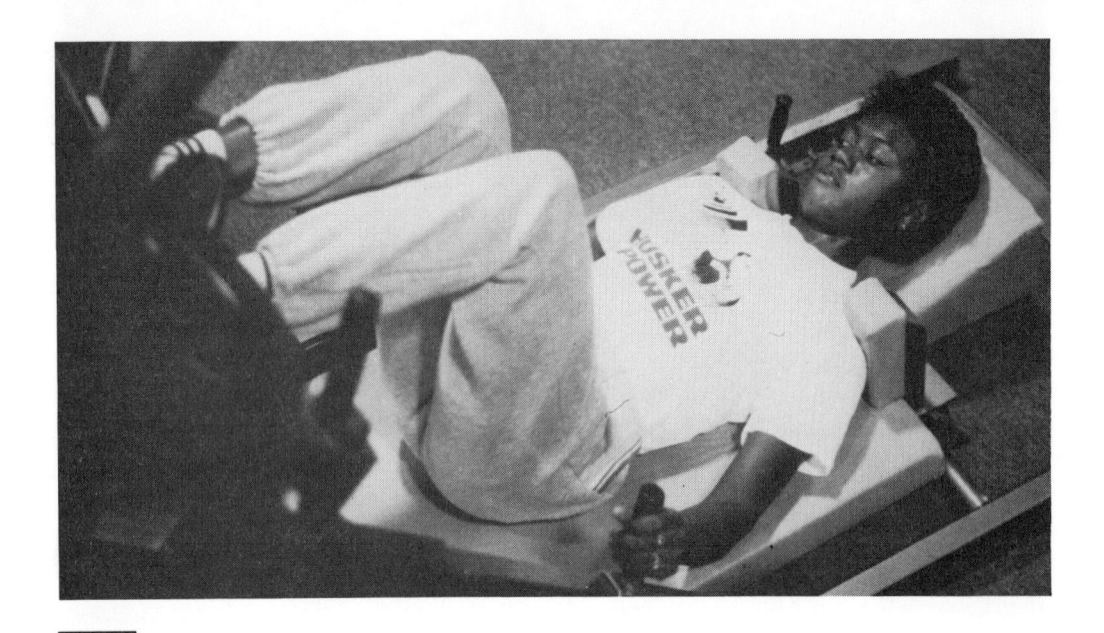

Figure 7.20
Hip Sled. Merlene Ottey develops sprinting power on the hip sled to set world records.

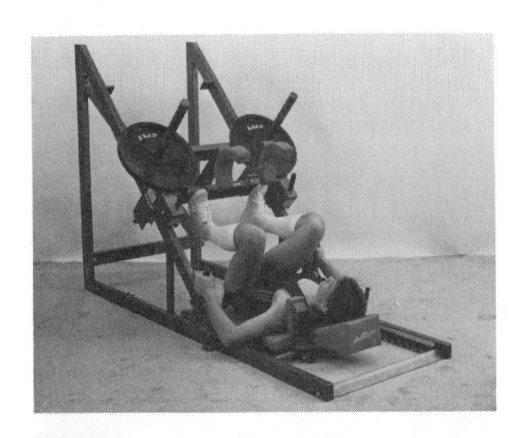

Figure 7.21
Hip Sled—Start

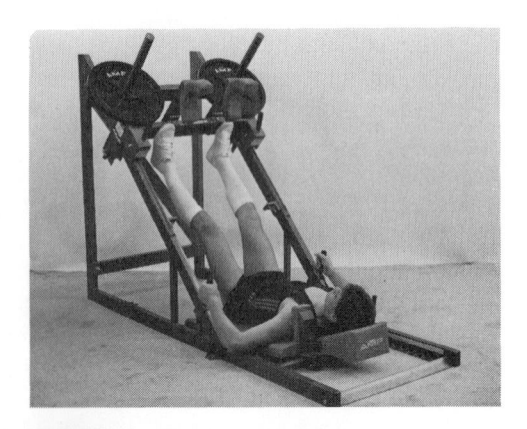

Figure 7.22
Hip Sled—Finish

Procedure Start on your back with the head and shoulders comfortably placed on hip sled board. Place feet the desired width apart on the foot rest. Make sure locking mechanism is engaged. To adjust the board forward, simply grasp the hip sled hand grips and pull the board forward. Each adjustment is 2 inches. A person 6 feet tall uses setting #7, 6 feet 2 inches uses setting #8, 5 feet 10 inches uses setting #6, and so on. (You need not get off the board to make this adjustment.) Position hands on the hip sled board hand grips. Move the carriage up the 45 degree angle track by extending your legs. Lower the carriage slowly and repeat.

Value This exercise will develop the quadriceps, hamstrings, and gluteus maximus muscles. This is a major exercise and can be used in place of the squat.

Equipment A hip sled is necessary for this exercise. The carriage by itself with no weights is 150 pounds.

Lunge

The lunge is a good exercise for leg development, especially for those of you who don't have a squat rack or a hip sled. The poundage used on the lunge is far less than the poundage used on the squat, which makes the lunge a much safer exercise. However, it is still a good idea to use the squat rack uprights to support the bar when doing the lunge. One spotter standing behind you is also a good idea. **Note:** If you don't have a squat rack for the bar to rest on, you should be able to clean and press the bar overhead and lower it onto your shoulders (just behind the neck) to perform the lunge. When finished, jerk the bar overhead and lower it to the ground by keeping the back straight and bending at the knees. Mike Rozier, 1983 Heisman Trophy winner was such a strong, natural athlete that since he already weighed 212 pounds he didn't really need the added size or added strength that he would have received from the squat exercise. So I had him concentrate on the lunge as his major leg exercise. Mike says,

> "The lunge will give you power to improve running speed. I recommend running backs start lifting in junior high school."

Mike Rozier was the UPI National Player of the Year. He won the Maxwell Award, was consensus All-American twice, and was UPI and AP Offensive Player of the Year twice, in addition to winning the Heisman Trophy.

Thousands of athletes were made aware of the benefits of this fine exercise when Mike Rozier was featured on a poster doing the lunge. The lunge is particularly good for anyone who wants to firm up his or her hips, so you might want to tell other members of your family about the lunge.

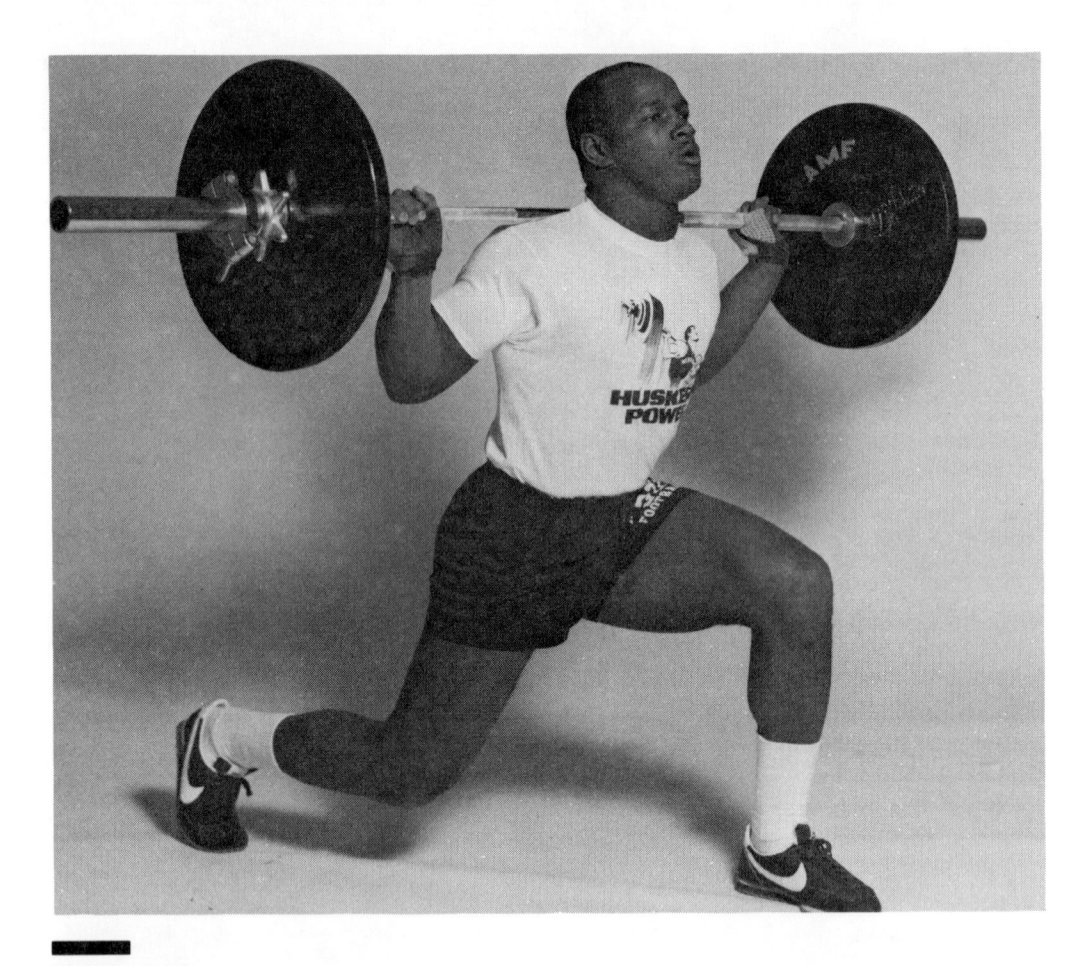

Figure 7.23
Lunge. 1983 Heisman Trophy winner, Mike Rozier, demonstrates the lunge.

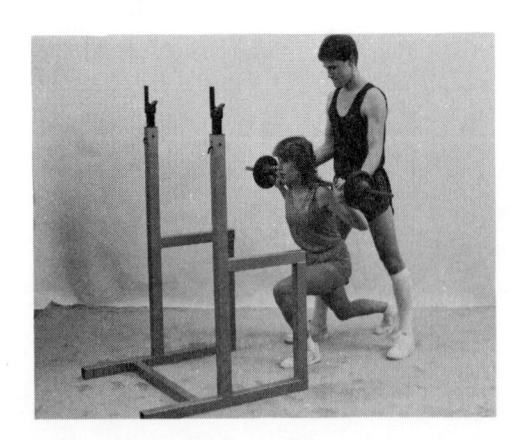

Figure 7.24
Lunge

Procedure The starting position is very similar to that of the squat, except the feet are closer together and are pointed straight ahead. Keeping the head up, step forward with the left foot about three feet so that the middle of the thigh is parallel with the ground, and lower yourself down into the lunge position, as shown. The right knee does not touch the ground. Extend the left leg, pushing against the ground to regain the starting position. Alternate legs and repeat.

Value This exercise will develop the quadriceps, hamstrings, and gluteus maximus, in addition to the vastus medialis in the knee area. This is generally a supplementary leg exercise; however, it could serve as a major exercise for you if you don't have a squat rack or hip sled.

Equipment An Olympic bar (or a standard bar) and squat rack or squat uprights will be needed for this exercise.

Safety You'll be surprised at how little weight you need for this exercise to be effective. Start with the bar only.

Supplementary Exercises for Lower Leg Development

Heel Raises (7:3A)

Procedure When doing heel raises, always extend upward as high as you can and as low as you can. This will allow you to go through a further range of motion and get a good stretch on the muscle. Do this exercise smoothly, not fast. A "burning" sensation should be felt in the calves. Heel raises should be performed from three different angles; toes straight, toes in, and toes out.

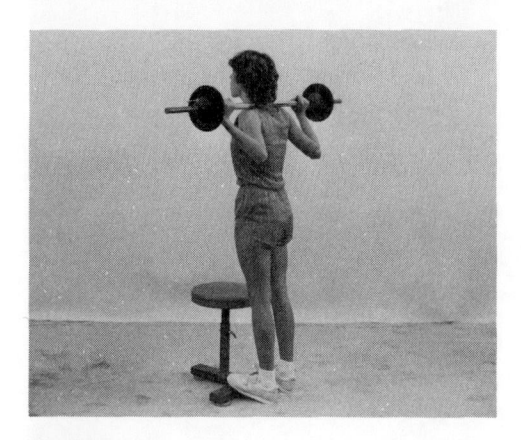

Figure 7.25
Heel Raises—Start

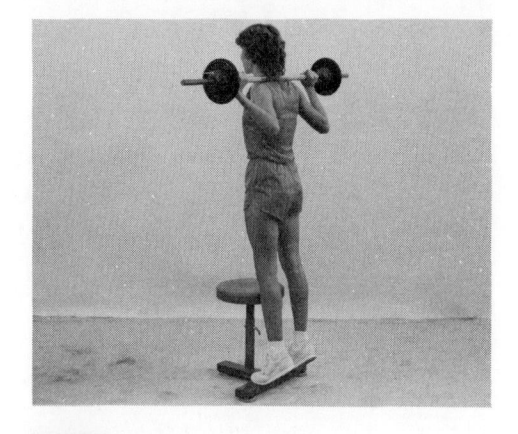

Figure 7.26
Heel Raises—Finish

Value This exercise will develop the gastrocnemius muscle (the calves) in the back of the lower leg. This is a supplementary leg exercise.

Equipment A barbell, a squat rack, and a two-by-four for a toe board (or AMF Squat Stool) are needed for this exercise.

Leg Extension (7:4)

If you have a leg extension apparatus, you should include this exercise in your program on Monday and Thursday. The leg extension exercise develops the muscle on the inside of your thigh, just above the knee. This muscle is called the vastus medialis. When this muscle is strong, it gives support to the stability of the knee joint. Its function is to extend the lower leg. Try sitting down in a chair with your knee bent, then extending your leg with your hand on the inside of your knee. You'll be able to feel this muscle work as it extends your leg. In the event that an athlete has injured the knee and has had knee surgery, strengthening this muscle is very important in regaining the stability of the knee joint. The leg extension is also important for the prevention of knee injuries. Sherri Hayward, All-American swimmer, tells why this is such an important exercise for her.

> "The leg extension exercise is a key source of leg strength for distance off the wall on the backstroke start. The added leg strength also gives me a powerful thrust on each of my turns. My strength program was a key ingredient in my success."

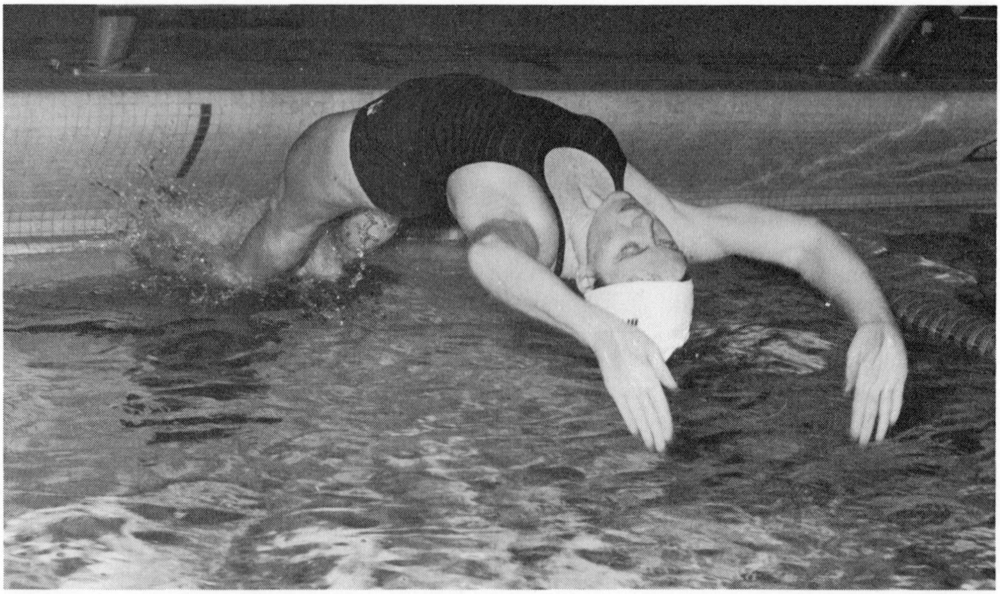

Figure 7.27
Sherri Hayward used her strength to gain All American honors three times.

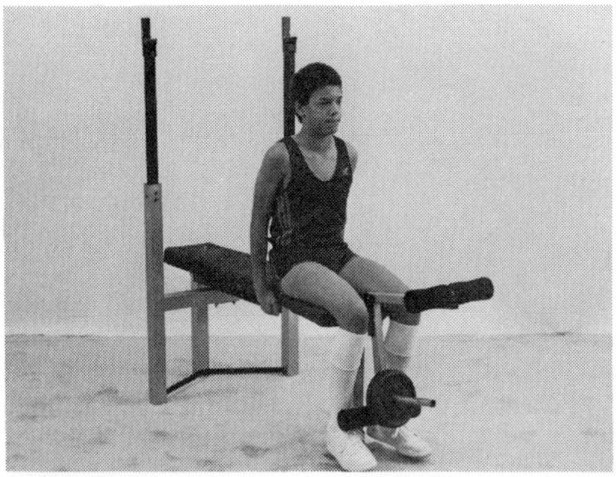

Figure 7.28
Leg Extension—Start

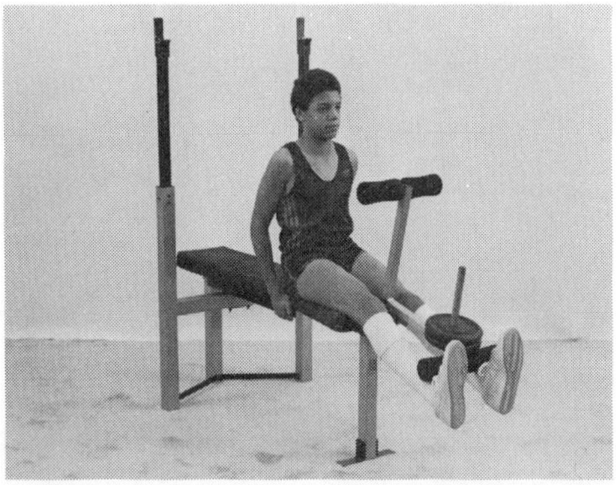

Figure 7.29
Leg Extension—Finish

Sherri worked extremely hard not only on her leg strength, but on her entire strength training program during her career at Nebraska. She was named All-Big-Eight four times and All-American three times.

Procedure While sitting on the end of your bench, hook the front of the ankle behind the roller pads. Slowly extend the lower leg outward until the leg is "locked out". Hold this position for a moment, and then lower the weight slowly and smoothly. When the weight is lowered, try to allow the weights to just barely touch, and then extend the lower leg outward again. This exercise should be performed slowly and smoothly so that you can "feel" the muscle working as you extend up and lower the weight.

Value This exercise will develop the vastus medialis on the inside front of the thigh. This is a major leg exercise for your program.

Equipment A leg extension machine, or attachment for your bench, are needed for this exercise. If you don't have a leg extension device, you may need to do this exercise at school or health club facility.

7:5 Leg Curl

If you have a leg curl apparatus, you should include this exercise along with the leg extension to supplement the major exercise you have chosen (squat, hip sled, or lunge). The leg curl exercise develops a muscle on the back of your thigh, called the hamstring. This muscle works in association with the front of the thigh in helping you to run and walk. Muscles come in pairs. One muscle in each pair helps contract your arm or leg, etc., while the other muscle in the pair helps you extend your arm or leg. As we develop these muscles through strength training, we must maintain a balance of strength so that one group of muscles doesn't get stronger than the other. Since we have selected a major exercise affecting the front of the thigh (squat, hip sled or lunge, as well as the leg extension), which works on the extension

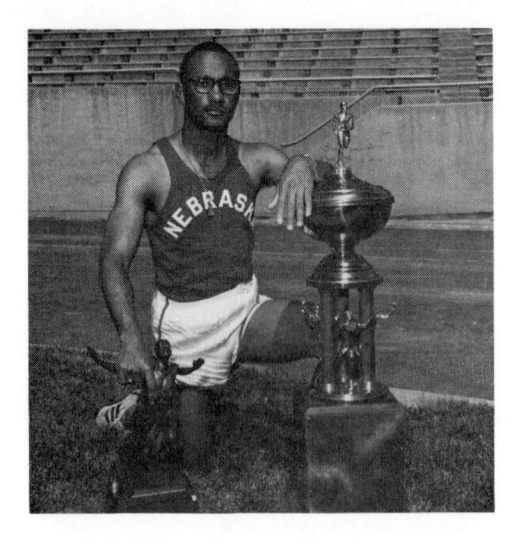

Figure 7.30
Charlie Greene was one of the greatest sprinters of all time.

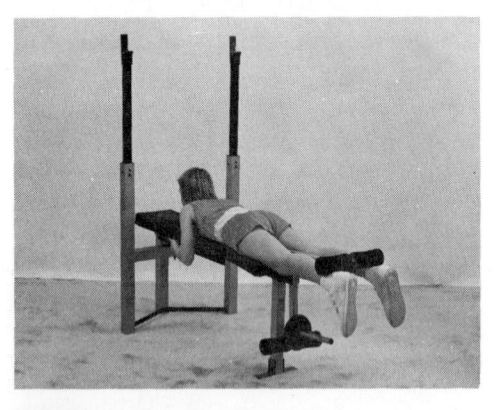

Figure 7.31
Leg Curl—Start

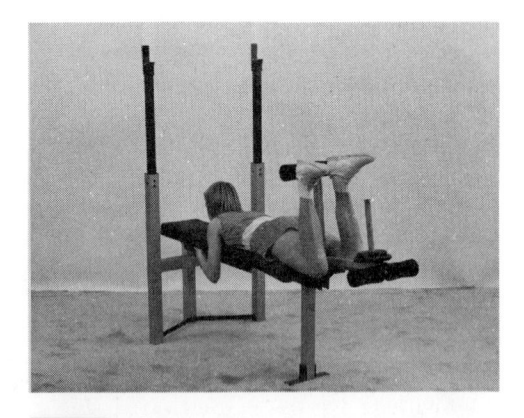

Figure 7.32
Leg Curl—Finish

of the leg, we then need to add an exercise to our program for the contraction of the leg. The leg curl exercise will strengthen the hamstring muscle, allowing the balance of strength to be maintained in your legs. Charlie Greene says, "The natural balance between the hamstring and the quadricep (thigh) must be monitored very closely. Therefore, I recommend lifting weights only under the direction of a qualified strength coach. Boyd Epley is one of the best."

Charlie Greene wasn't just another great Nebraska athlete; he was one of the greatest sprinters in United States history. Charlie won both the NCAA and Big Eight 100-yard dash championships three years in a row, and was named the outstanding athlete in the prestigious Big Eight Conference three times in a row. He has held several world records, and was an Olympic gold and bronze medallist in the 1968 Olympic Games in Mexico City. Charlie and Johnny Rodgers used to work legs together. They both took leg development very seriously.

Procedure While lying in the prone position (on your stomach) hook the ankles under the roller pads while keeping the hips on the bench. Slowly curl the lower leg toward the buttocks as far as you can; hold it for a moment and then lower the weight slowly. When the weight is lowered, try to allow the weights to just barely touch, and then curl the weight again. Do this exercise slowly and smoothly so you can feel the muscle working as you flex and lower the weight.

Value This exercise will develop the hamstrings (the back of the thigh). This is a major exercise in your program. This exercise should be included in your program to help balance out the development to the front of the thigh.

Equipment A leg curl machine, or an attachment on your bench press bench, is needed for this exercise. If you don't have a leg curl device you may need to do this exercise at school or a health club facility.

Recommended Exercises for the Stomach

Incline Sit-up (7:6)

Sometime during your athletic career you may see an athlete vomit after exerting an all-out effort in a race. Many times it is because the stomach muscles are not used to being contracted that many times in such a short period of time. Exercises for the stomach are many times overlooked in a lifting program. Strengthening the stomach by doing repeated contractions, such as sit-ups, allows you to condition the stomach for a greater work load, and

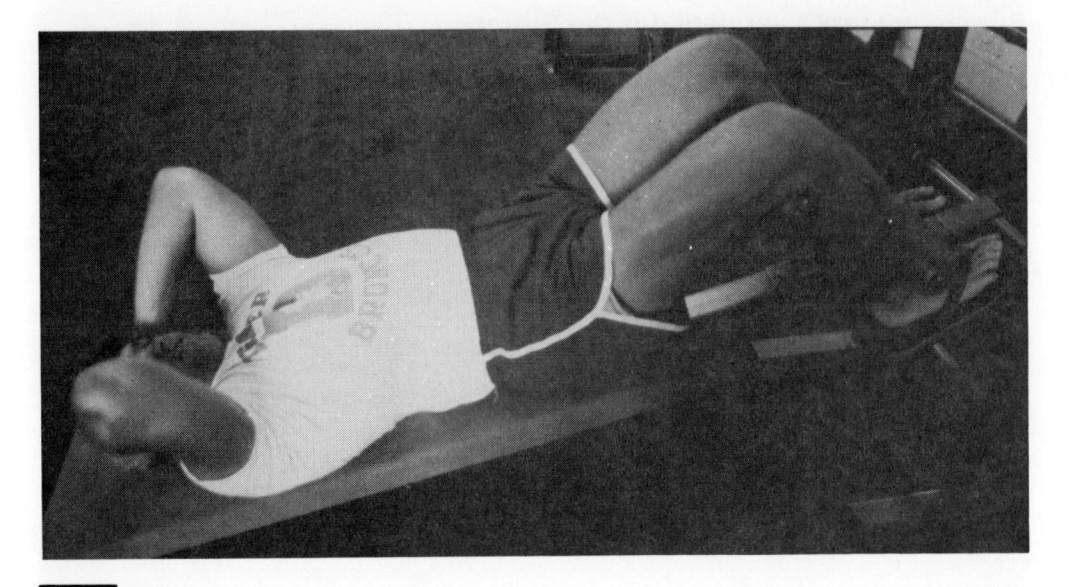

Figure 7.33
Kelvin Clark demonstrates the incline sit-up.

Monday–Thursday Lifting Exercises

in most cases will prevent the unpleasant experience of vomiting. Kelvin Clark is a 260-pound offensive guard, formerly with the Denver Broncos, who now plays for the New Orleans Saints. Kelvin is shown doing the incline sit-up exercise. The sit-up was one of Kelvin's favorite exercises during his college days. In fact, he tripled the number of sit-ups he could do in a one month period.

Kelvin was 215 pounds coming out of high school in Odessa, Texas. He had never lifted with barbells before, so he was able to manage only 170 pounds for twelve repetitions on the bench press. He did his program as outlined, and I used to work out with him myself because he was intense and worked hard. As a senior he bench pressed 400 pounds, and weighed 274 pounds. He was named All-American and also made the All-American Strength Team.

Kelvin says, "I have always included sit-ups in my program. I used to have contests with other players to see who could do the most in 30 seconds. Young athletes should not overlook stomach work in their program."

Procedure Whether you use a sit-up board or lie on the floor, be sure to keep your knees bent and the hands behind the head. As you sit up, concentrate on the abdominal muscles "pulling" the upper body upward. For best results do this exercise smoothly and slowly.

Value This exercise will develop the abdominal muscles (stomach). This is considered a major exercise for the stomach.

Equipment An AMF Adjustable Incline Sit-Up Board may be used to increase the difficulty of this exercise.

Safety Bend the knees when doing sit-ups to reduce strain on the lower back.

Supplementary Exercises for the Stomach

7:6A Crunch   7:6D Jackknife

7:6B Side bend   7:6E Trunk twist

7:6C Knee-up

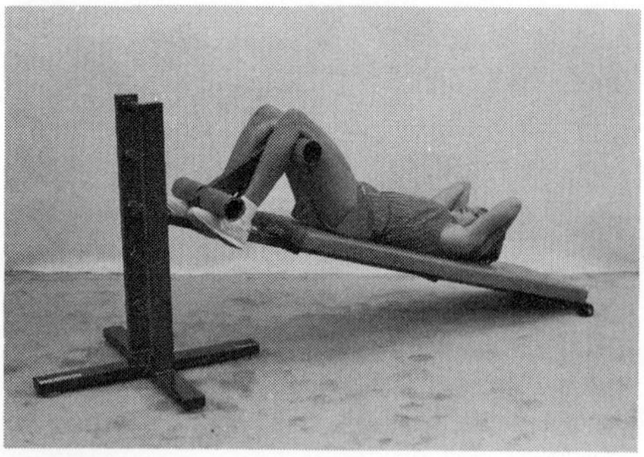

Figure 7.34
Incline Sit-Up—Start

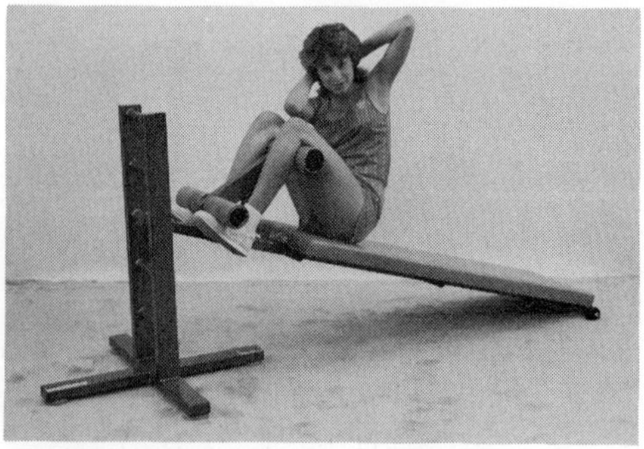

Figure 7.35
Incline Sit-Up—Finish

Crunch (7:6A)

Procedure While lying on the back, slightly spread the legs, clasp hands behind the head, and lift the head off the floor four to six inches. Hold this position for a pause. Then pull yourself up to twelve to eighteen inches from the floor, and hold for a moment. Return to the lower position, hold for a pause, and then lie flat. Repeat. When you can do no more, spread the legs and lift the right leg six inches off the ground. Place both hands on the right leg. Slide the hands up the leg until they reach the knee. Keep the legs spread, your leg a constant six inches high, and the hands reaching toward the outside of the knee. Switch legs and repeat.

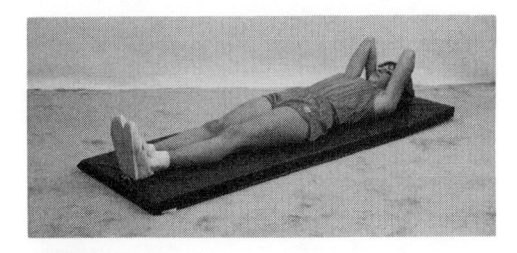

Figure 7.36
Crunch—Start

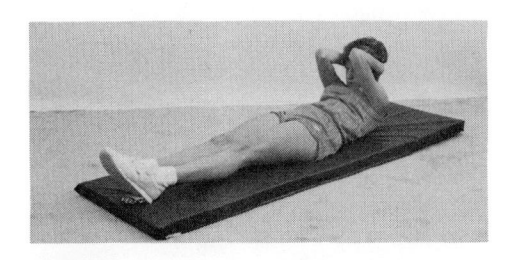

Figure 7.37
Crunch—#2 Position

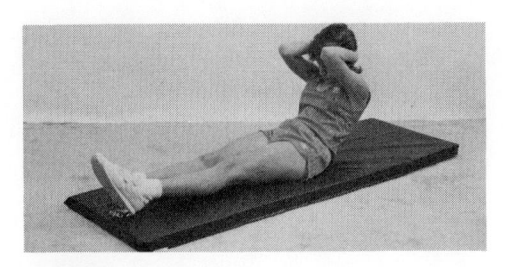

Figure 7.38
Crunch—#3 Position

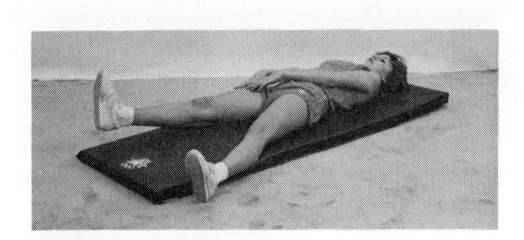

Figure 7.39
Crunch—Position #4

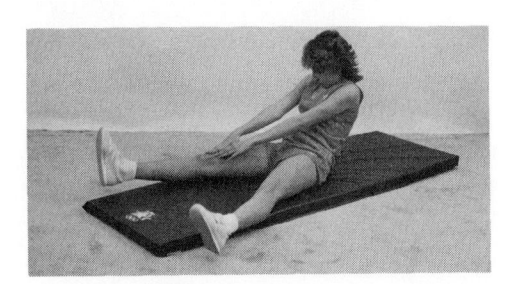

Figure 7.40
Crunch—Position #5

Monday–Thursday Lifting Exercises

Value This exercise will develop the external abdominal obliques (the sides of your waist) and the rectus abdominals (the middle of your stomach). This is a supplemental exercise that should require fewer sets than recommended for major exercises. This exercise could be included in your program as a substitute for the incline sit-up.

Equipment None.

Side Bend (7:6B)

Procedure Hold a dumbbell in the right hand while the feet are about six inches apart. Slide the left hand down the left leg until the knee is touched. After the knee is touched, lower the right hand (the one with the dumbbell) down the right leg as far as you can. Do not allow the upper body to sway as you move from side to side. After a set with the right hand, switch the dumbbell to the left hand immediately.

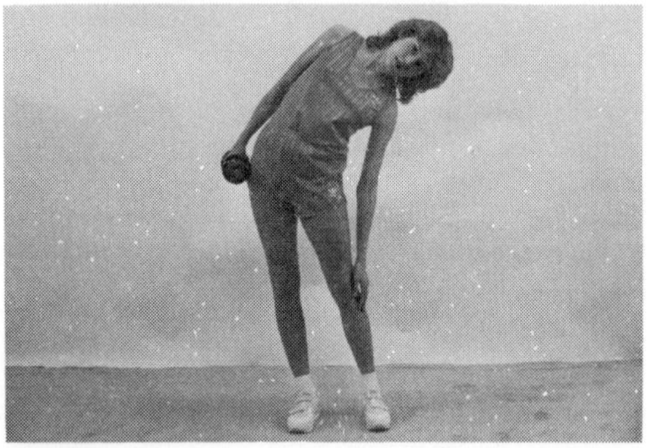

Figure 7.41
Side Bend—Start

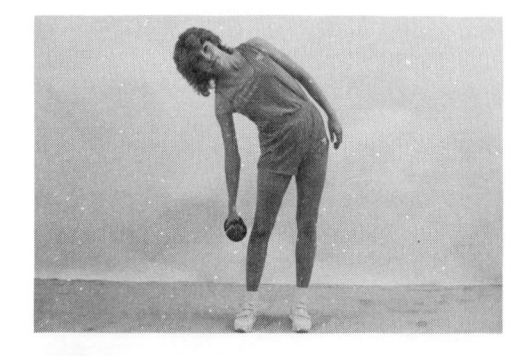

Figure 7.42
Side Bend—Finish

Value This exercise will develop the external abdominal oblique muscles (the sides of your waist). This is a supplementary stomach exercise.

Equipment Dumbbells.

Knee-Up (7:6C)

Procedure Lie on your back, extend the legs outward and reach in the opposite direction with the arms. Keep the legs, arms, and head off the floor at all times. At the same time, pull the knees up toward the trunk, and sit up with the upper body as the arms reach out past the legs. Return to the starting position and repeat. It may take several workouts to develop coordination for this exercise. This exercise should be done quickly.

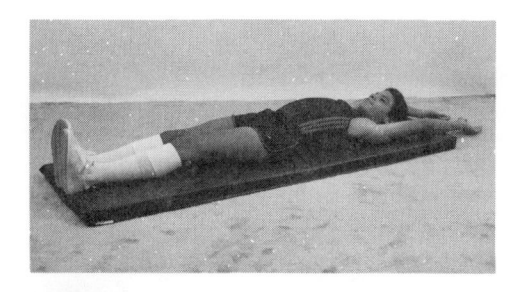

Figure 7.43
Knee-Up—Start

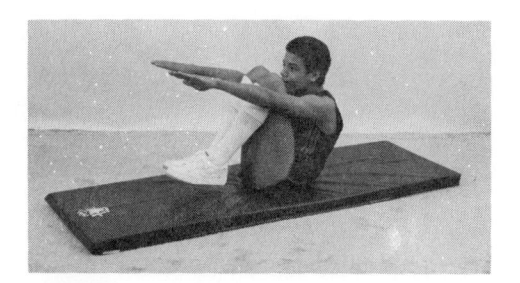

Figure 7.44
Knee-Up—Finish

Value This exercise will develop both the upper and lower portions of the mid-section. This is listed as a supplementary exercise, however it could serve as a substitute for the incline sit-up.

Equipment Sit-up mat or carpet.

Jackknife (7:6D)

Procedure The jackknife is very similar to the knee-up. The starting position is the same. In place of bending the knees and pulling them towards the upper body, keep the legs straight as the upper body sits up. The jackknife should be done quickly.

Value This exercise will develop the abdominal muscles of the mid-section. This is listed as a supplementary exercise, however it could serve as a substitute for the incline sit-up.

Equipment Sit-up mat or carpet.

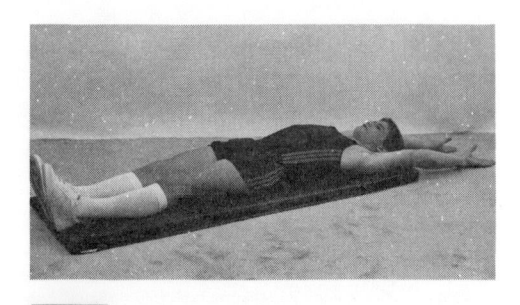

Figure 7.45
Jackknife—Start

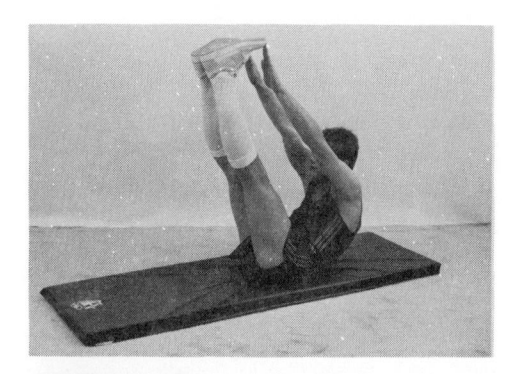

Figure 7.46
Jackknife—Finish

Trunk Twist (7:6E)

Procedure Place a broomstick across the back of the shoulders and place the hands out wide as you are sitting on a bench. While keeping the hips motionless, twist the upper body all the way to the left and then to the right; repeat the twisting. This exercise should be done quickly.

Value This exercise will develop the external abdominal oblique muscles (sides of the waist). This is a supplementary exercise.

Equipment A broomstick and your bench.

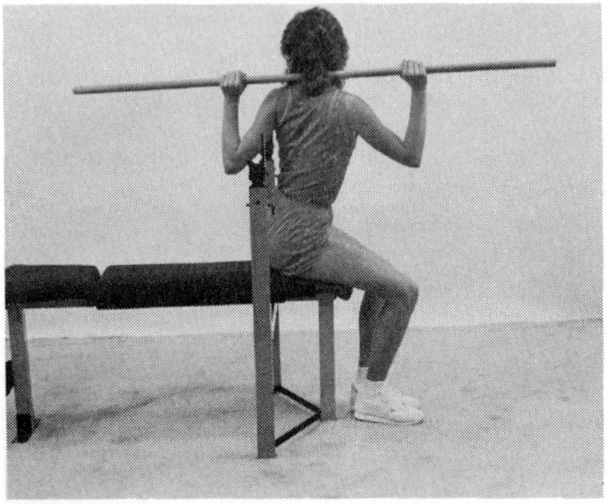

Figure 7.47
Trunk Twist—Start

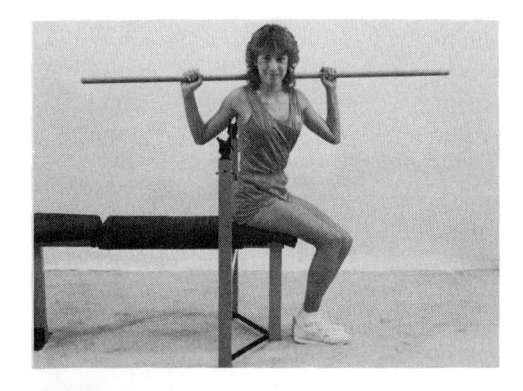

Figure 7.48
Trunk Twist—Finish

CHAPTER EIGHT

Tuesday-Friday Lifting Exercises

This chapter presents the six exercises that are most important for your back, shoulder, and arm development. These six exercises are to be performed on Tuesday and again on Friday of each week in your off-season program.

1. Upright row
2. Military press
3. Lateral raise
4. Bent-over raise
5. Curl
6. Tricep extension

In addition to the six major exercises are several supplementary exercises. Along with the exercises are comments from successful (and famous) athletes who have realized the value of the Tuesday-Friday lifting program.

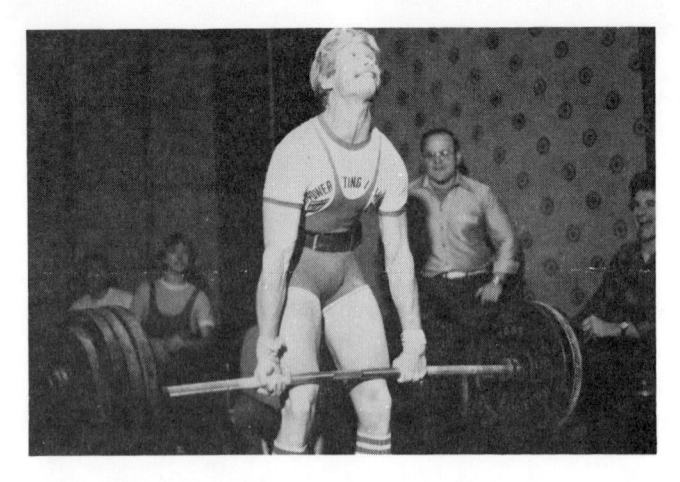

Figure 8.1
Mike Arthur Sets World Record

Recommended Exercises for the Back

Upright row (8:1)

You should be doing the upright row exercise at this time for your back development, with plans to do the power clean exercise in the future. The power clean is an advanced exercise, and not recommended for the young athlete, and is therefore not presented in this book. Mike Arthur says, "The young athlete needs strength in the upper body to be competitive in athletics, especially young girls. The upright row exercise will develop the trapezius muscles of your upper back." Mike Arthur is a former world recordholder in powerlifting. He

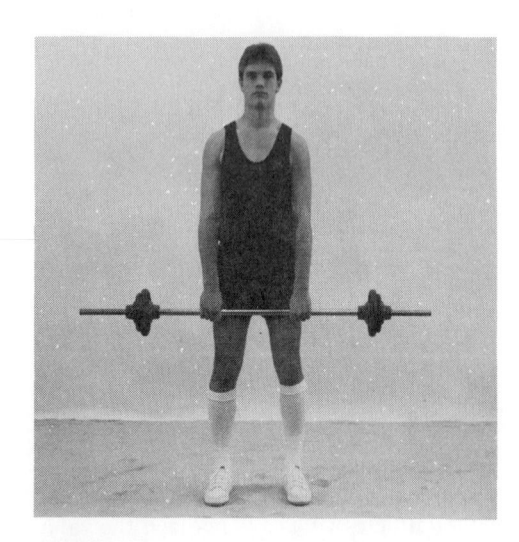

Figure 8.2
Upright Row—Start

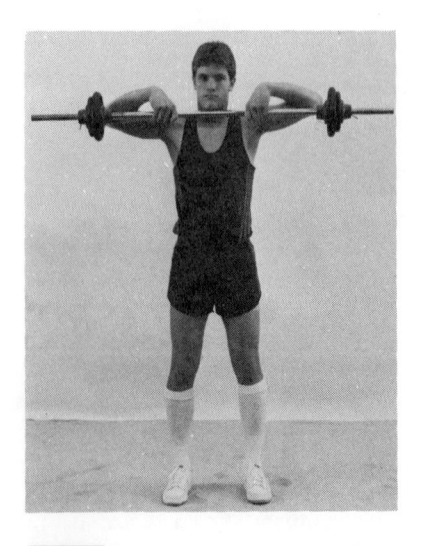

Figure 8.3
Upright Row—Finish

was the national collegiate champion and won the Nebraska state powerlifting championships ten years in a row. Mike says, "Even though I set a world record in the Deadlift, I don't recommend the deadlift for athletes. The power clean is a much more explosive exercise and much better for developing the power necessary for athletics. The upright row is a good substitute for the power clean and will provide good back development for the young athlete."

Procedure From a standing position, hold the bar at arm's length, hands four to eight inches apart, using an overhand grip. Pull the bar up to the chin as the elbows are pulled outward and upward. Lower the bar to arm's length and repeat. The bar should be kept close to the body at all times. This exercise should be done slowly and smoothly.

Value This exercise will develop the trapezius muscle of the upper back and neck region. This is a recommended major back exercise for the young athlete.

Equipment: Barbell.

Supplementary Exercises for Back Development

8:1A Shoulder shrug   8:1D Dumbbell row

8:1B Hyperextension   8:1E Pullover

8:1C Bent-over row

Shoulder Shrug (8:1A)

Procedure From a standing position hold the bar at arm's length. Elevate the shoulders, as if you are trying to touch your ears, and then pull them back, down, and forward in a circular fashion. Hold the bar for a moment at its peak and then continue with the circular movement. This exercise should be done slowly and smoothly. The shoulder shrug may also be

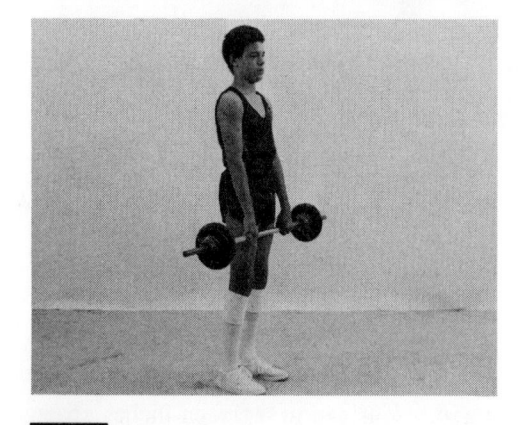

Figure 8.4
Shoulder Shrug—Start

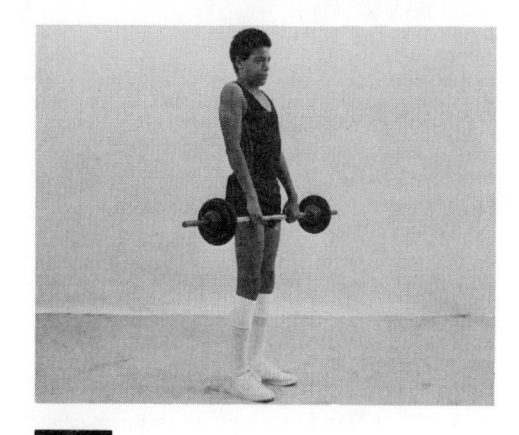

Figure 8.5
Shoulder Shrug—Finish

performed with dumbbells. Dumbbell shrugs may allow for a slightly greater range of motion due to the fact that they are independent of each other, and because there is not a problem with the bar hitting the legs.

Value This exercise will develop the trapezius muscle (upper back). This exercise is a supplementary back exercise.

Equipment A barbell or dumbbells can be used for this exercise.

Hyperextension (8:1B)

Procedure The upper body should be hanging straight down. From this position extend the upper body upward. As the body is raised upward, the elbows should flare out. This exercise should be performed slowly and smoothly.

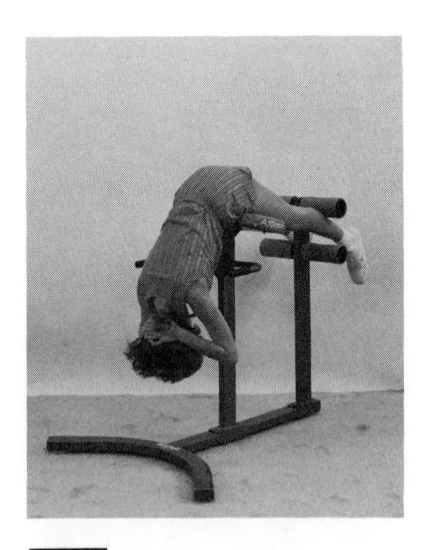

Figure 8.6
Hyperextension—Start

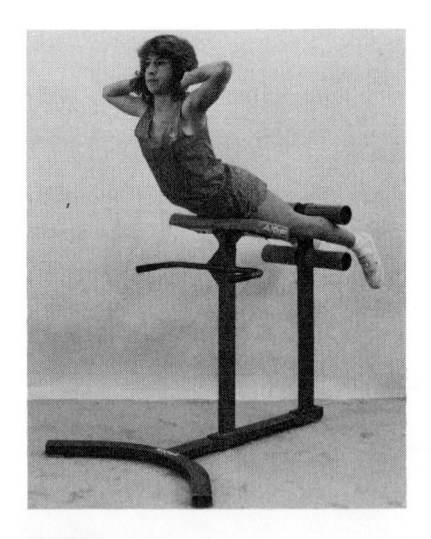

Figure 8.7
Hyperextension—Finish

Value This exercise will develop the spinal erectors of the lower back.

Equipment A hyperextension bench is needed for this exercise.

Bent-Over Row (8:1C)

Procedure Bending over from the waist, slightly bend the knees, and hold the bar at arm's length. The hands should be in an overhand grip about fourteen to eighteen inches apart. The bar should be about one to two inches off the floor when starting the exercise. Pull the bar into the waist as the elbows are pulled upward and slightly outward. This exercise should be performed slowly and smoothly.

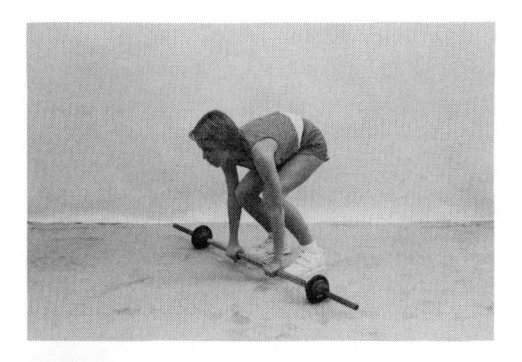

Figure 8.8
Bent-Over Row—Start

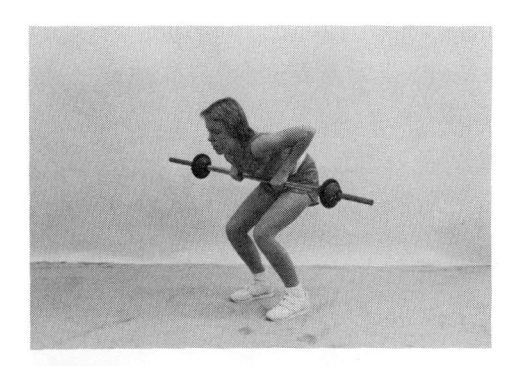

Figure 8.9
Bent-Over Row—Finish

Value This exercise will develop the latissimus dorsi muscle.

Equipment A standard bar may be used for this exercise.

Safety A slight bend in the knees should prevent any strain on the back of the leg, and also provide greater stability.

Dumbbell Bent-Over Row (8:1D)

Procedure Bend over from the waist, slightly bend the knees, and hold the dumbbell at arm's length. The dumbbell should be about one to two inches off the floor when starting the exercise. While leaning on a stool or workbench, pull the dumbbell up as high as possible, then lower and repeat. This exercise should be performed slowly and smoothly.

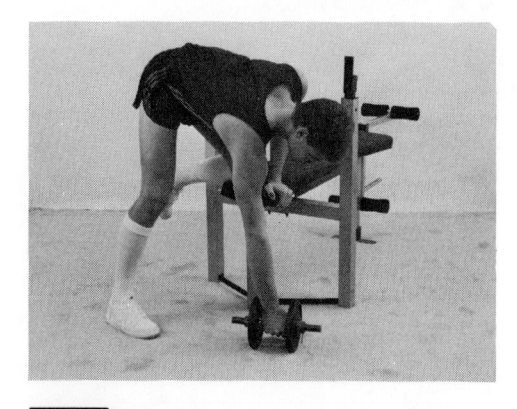

Figure 8.10
Dumbbell Row—Start

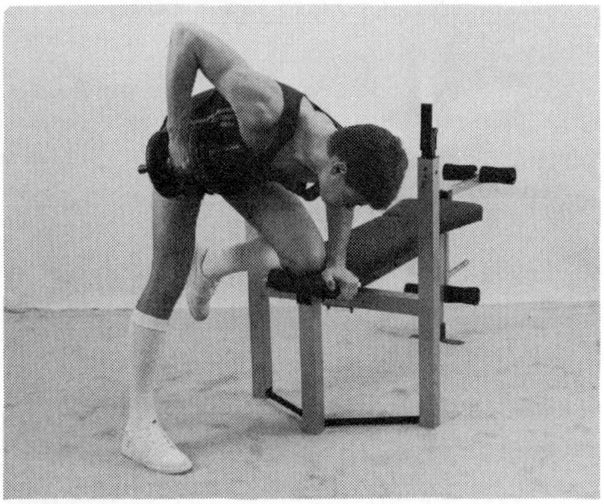

Figure 8.11
Dumbbell Row—Finish

Tuesday–Friday Lifting Exercises   89

Value This exercise will develop the latissimus dorsi muscle.

Equipment The dumbbell is needed for this exercise, as well as a bench or a stool for support.

Pullover (8:1E)

Procedure Lie on your back on the bench while holding the bar on the chest. Keep the bend in the elbows as you push the bar over the head, and as the bar is lowered to the floor. Allow the weight to just barely touch the floor, and then pull the bar upward and over the head. The head should be kept on the bench, and the bar should come within two to four inches of the head. This exercise should be performed slowly and smoothly.

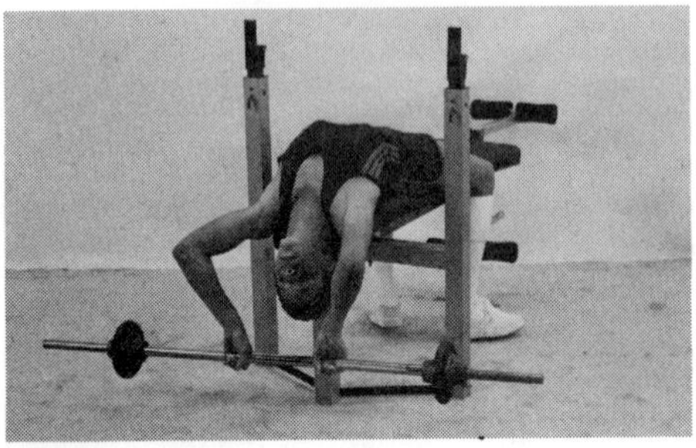

Figure 8.12
Pull-Over—Start

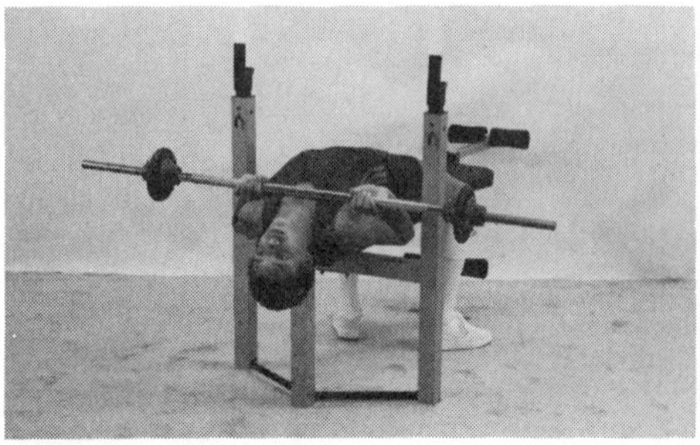

Figure 8.13
Pull-Over—Finish

Value This exercise will develop the latissimus dorsi and the small serratus anterior muscles located between the ribs.

Equipment A standard barbell and bench.

Recommended Exercises for the Shoulders
Military Press (8:2)

This exercise will develop the front of your shoulders. The shoulder muscle is called the deltoid. The deltoid muscle of your shoulder is made up of three parts: the anterior, or the front; the medial, or the middle; and the posterior, or the back.

Vince Ferragamo was not the typical fragile quarterback. He was one of the strongest and most durable quarterbacks in Nebraska football history. He was All-American in 1976, and led the Los Angeles Rams to the 1980 Super Bowl. Vince says, "Shoulder work has given me the added strength I need to throw deep and the confidence to block and tackle when I need to. Young athletes should not overlook their shoulder exercises".

Procedure Use an overhand grip with the hands about fifteen to twenty inches apart. Press the bar overhead, lower the bar to the upper chest, and repeat. Try to keep the elbows pointed forward. This exercise should be performed slowly and smoothly, and can be performed either standing or seated.

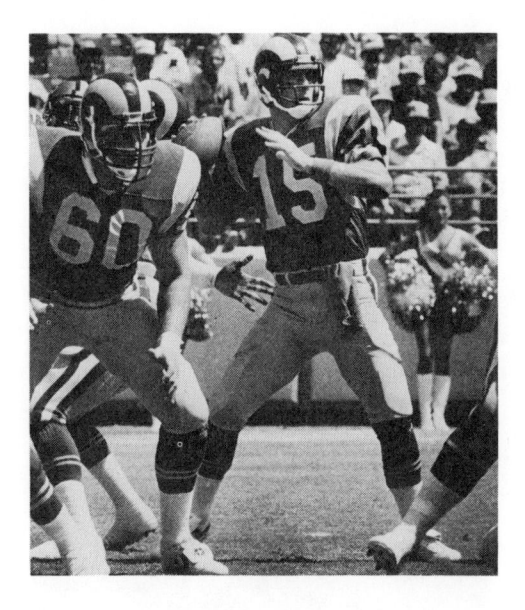

Figure 8.14
Vince Ferragamo Throws Deep for L.A.

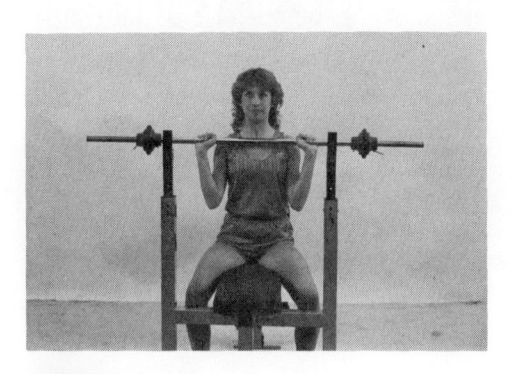

Figure 8.15
Military Press—Start

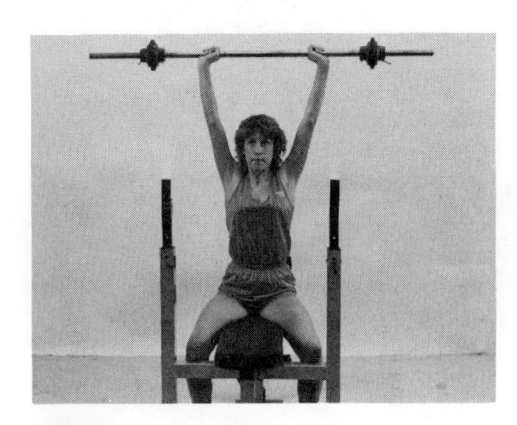

Figure 8.16
Military Press—Finish

Value This exercise will develop the anterior deltoid (front of the shoulder).

Equipment A barbell and squat rack are needed if done standing. A barbell and bench are needed if done seated.

Safety A supportive lumbar lifting belt is recommended for this exercise.

Supplementary Exercises for the Military Press

       8:2A Behind the neck press

       8:2B Dumbbell shoulder press

Tuesday–Friday Lifting Exercises   91

Behind the Neck Press (8:2A)

Procedure Place the bar behind the neck with an overhand grip about the same width as for your bench press. This exercise should be performed from a sitting position. This sitting position will not allow as much overall body movement as standing. The bar should be resting on the upper back. Press the bar overhead, and keep the elbows pointed outward. Lower the bar and repeat the exercise. This exercise should be performed slowly and smoothly.

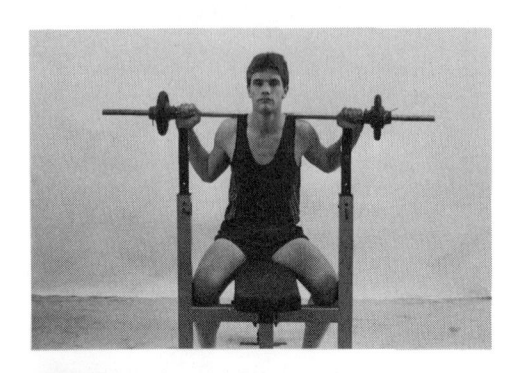

Figure 8.17
Behind-the-Neck Press—Start

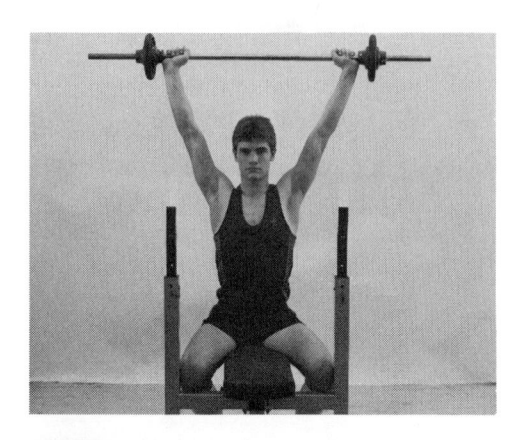

Figure 8.18
Behind-the-Neck Press—Finish

Value This exercise will develop the anterior deltoid (front of shoulder). This could serve as a major exercise in place of the military press for your program.

Equipment A barbell and free standing shoulder press seat are best; however, your bench can be used.

Safety A supportive lumbar lifting belt is recommended for this exercise.

Dumbbell Shoulder Press (8:2B)

Procedure This exercise can be performed standing or sitting. Start with the dumbbells at the chest level position, with the palms facing away from the body. Press the right dumbbell upward until the arm is just short of locking out. Lower the dumbbell, and then press the left dumbbell upward. Lower the dumbbell and repeat. This exercise should be performed slowly and smoothly. The exercise can also be performed by pressing both dumbbells at the same time.

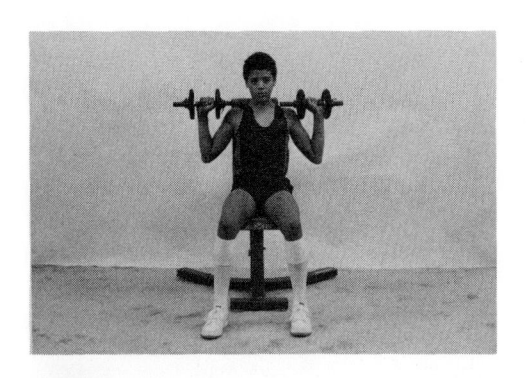

Figure 8.19
Dumbbell Shoulder Press—
Start

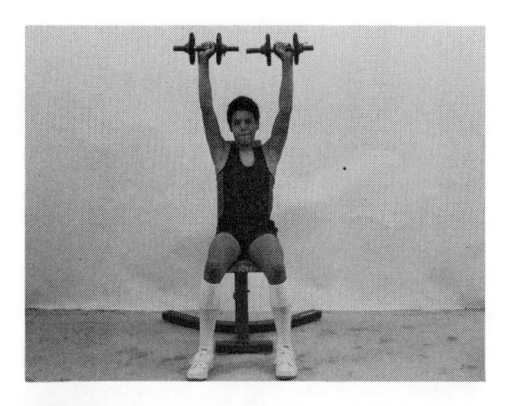

Figure 8.20
Dumbbell Shoulder Press—
Finish

Value This exercise will develop the anterior deltoid (front of the shoulder).

Equipment A pair of dumbbells is needed for this exercise, and if done in a seated position, a shoulder press seat or bench will also be needed.

Lateral Raise (8:3)

This exercise will develop the middle portion of the shoulder (the medial deltoid). Dumbbells are used to develop strength in each side of the body. The dumbbells also develop stabilizers that help balance the dumbbell from side to side, in addition to back and forth, as they are lifted up and down. Peggy Liddick was one of the strongest young women I have ever worked with. Peggy was a Big Eight champion gymnast herself, and is now head coach of the Nebraska School of Gymnastics. Her coaching has prepared many of the gymnasts for Francis Allen's teams at Nebraska, who have won the NCAA championship an unprecedented five years in a row. Peggy Liddick says,

> "Balanced shoulder development is essential in gymnastics. Three times a week our drills are geared toward shoulder strength."

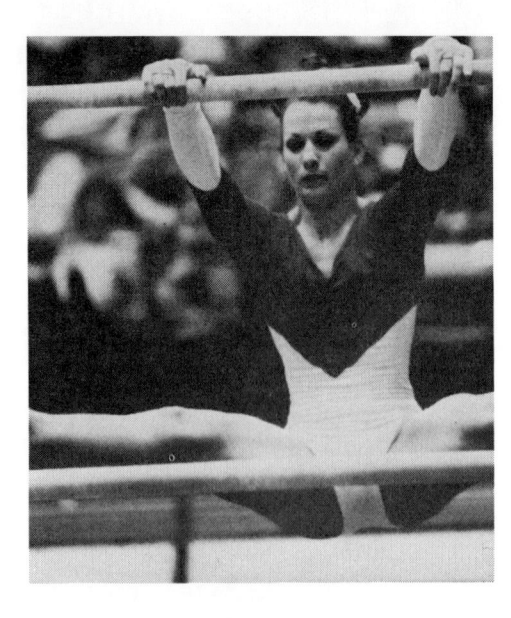

Figure 8.21
Peggy Liddick demonstrates her strength on the uneven bar.

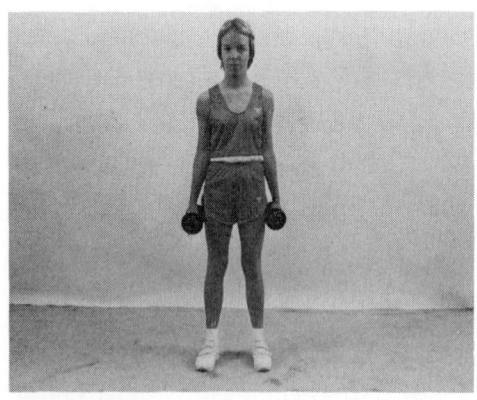

Figure 8.22
Lateral Raise—Start

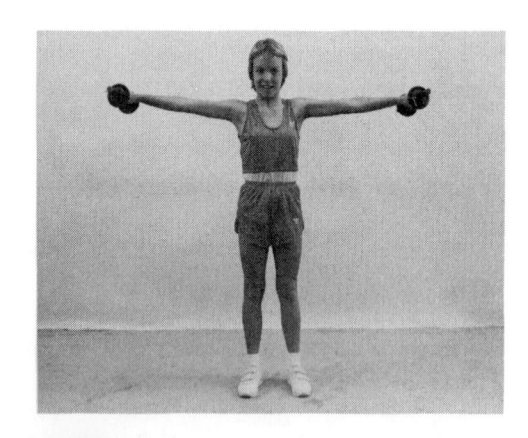

Figure 8.23
Lateral Raise—Finish

Procedure From the starting position, place the dumbbells by your side with the palms of your hands toward the legs. From this position, raise the dumbbells to the side laterally until the dumbbells are slightly above the shoulder joint. Use an overhead grip. There should be a very slight bend in the elbows so that some of the stress is not on the elbow joint. Lower the dumbbells and repeat.

Value This exercise will develop the medial deltoid (middle of shoulder).

Equipment Dumbbells are required.

Bent-Over Raise (8:4)

This exercise will develop the back portion of the shoulder, or the posterior deltoid. Many schools have a sixteen-station multipurpose exercise machine and use this machine for the military press to develop the front of athletes shoulders. Unless the school provides dumbbells in their program, the students do not have the opportunity to do the bent-over raise and, therefore, do not achieve balanced development in the shoulder. I have seen many athletes with the front part of their shoulders developed from pressing movements, but no development to the back of the shoulder. Don't let this happen to you. The back of your shoulder is important in performing many of the functions used in athletics. Jim Scherr says, "This exercise is especially helpful for wrestlers. When you do a sit-out move, strength in back of the shoulder will help you get your arm in proper position to make the move." Jim was the 1984 NCAA Wrestling Champion at 177 pounds. His twin brother was the 1984 champion at 190 pounds. The Scherr twins are your All-American-boy types. They don't smoke; they don't drink; and they are very religious. They compete in the classroom just as fiercely as they do on the wrestling mat or in the weight room. Jim is a three-time academic All-Big Eight wrestler, and Bill has been honored four times. Bill Scherr says, "In the off-season I follow the six week cycle program, and during the season I do two sets of ten repetitions. This program has really helped me."

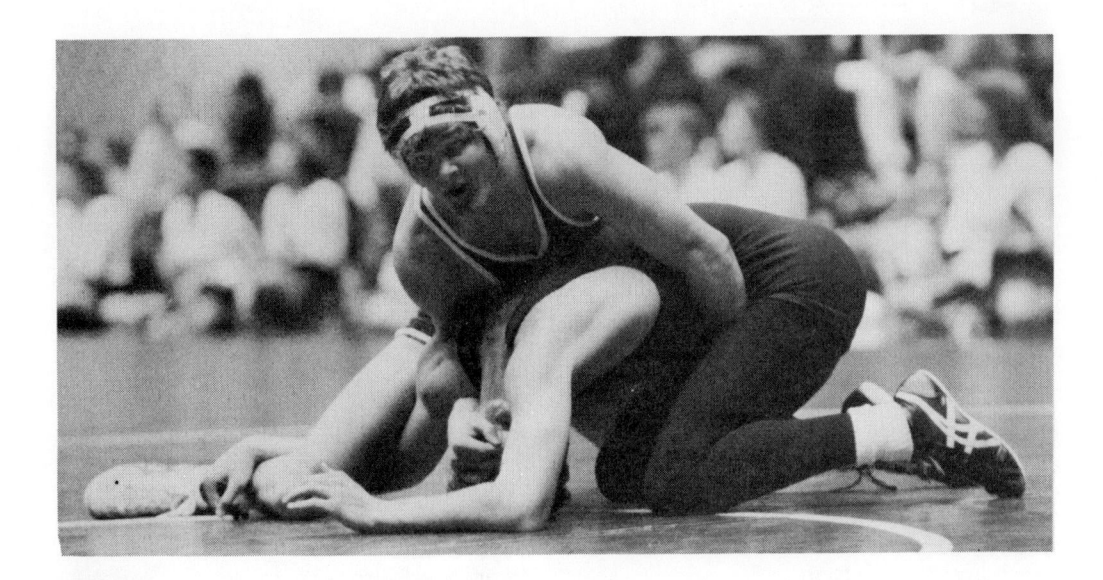

Figure 8.24
Jim Scherr was 1984 NCAA Champion at 177 pounds.

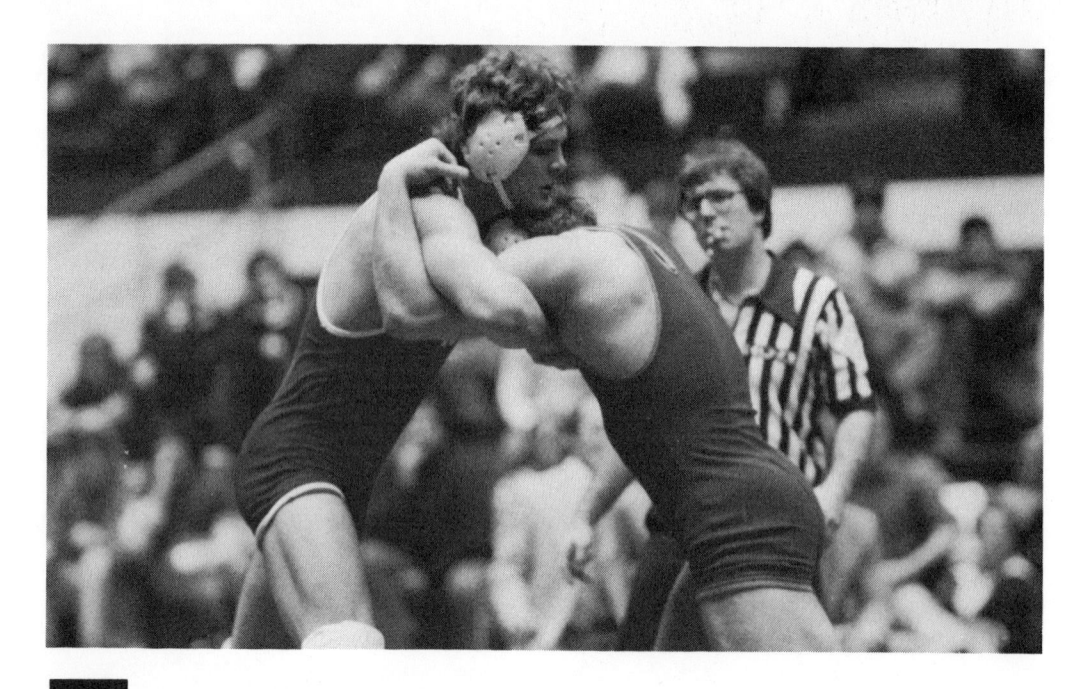

Figure 8.25
Bill Scherr was 1984 NCAA Champion at 190 pounds

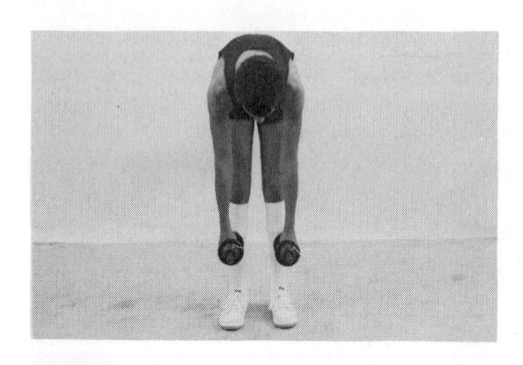

Figure 8.26
Bent-Over Raise—Start

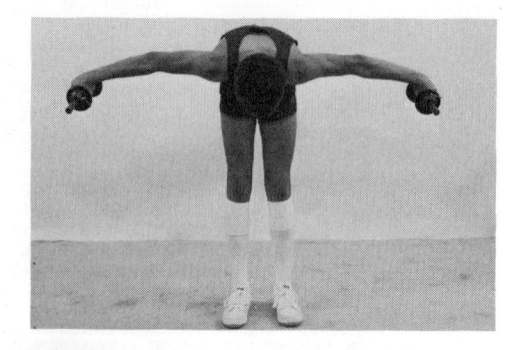

Figure 8.27
Bent-Over Raise—Finish

Procedure Bend forward from the waist with a slight bend in the knees. The arms should be hanging straight down with the palms facing each other. From this position, raise the dumbbells to the side and upward as far as possible. Lift the dumbbells together; lower and repeat. This lift should be performed slowly and smoothly, both on the up and downward movement.

Value This exercise will develop the posterior deltoid (back of shoulder). This exercise should be included in your program.

Equipment Dumbbells are required.

Safety A slight bend in the knees will prevent stress to the hamstring, and provide better balance.

Recommended Exercises for the Arms

Curl (8:5)

This exercise will develop the front of the upper arm, or the bicep. Some coaches discourage young athletes from doing the curl because it develops the bicep, which is not a major muscle in improvement of athletic performance like your chest and legs are. But, if you want a balanced program, I recommend that you include the curl exercise because, as discussed in

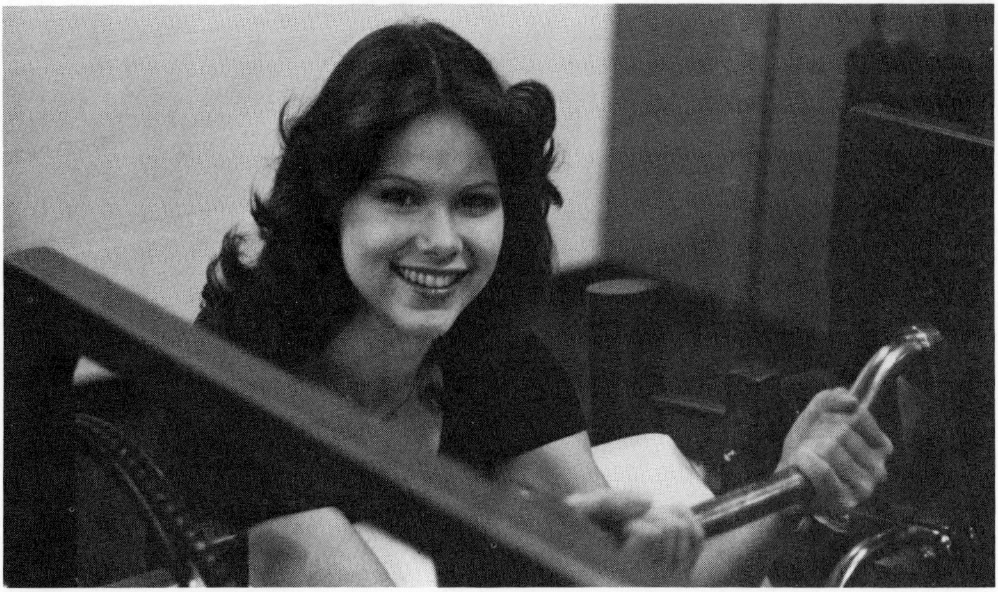

Figure 8.28
Guylyn Remmenga prepares herself for the Miss America Pageant.

Tuesday–Friday Lifting Exercises

Figure 8.29
Curl—Start

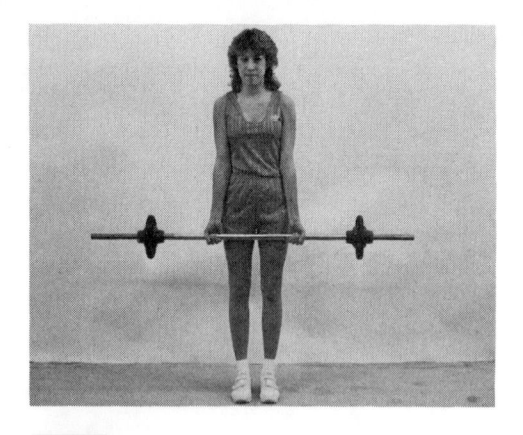

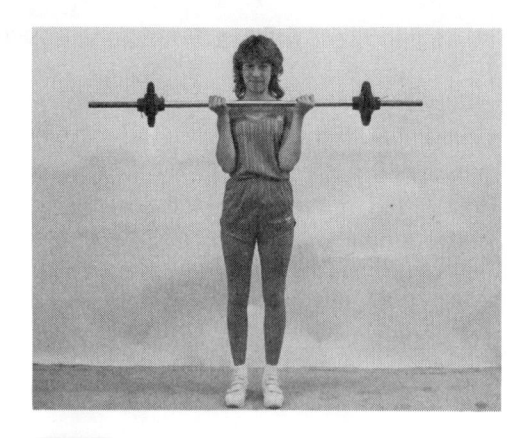

Figure 8.30
Curl—Finish

a previous chapter, your body's muscles work in pairs. The bicep in the front of your arm contracts your arm, while the tricep muscle in the back of your arm works to extend the arm. The two muscles work as a pair. You will want to have at least one exercise in your program for the bicep, and one for its counterpart, the tricep. A balanced program is important to many people, not just young athletes. Guylyn Remmenga, who was Miss Nebraska in 1978, asked me for a balanced program to help prepare her for the Miss America Pageant. Guylyn was very talented; in fact, she won the talent portion of the 1978 Miss America Pageant. What she needed was a balanced lifting program to give her more confidence in the swimsuit competition. Guylyn worked very hard in the weight room. (She is pictured in figure 8.28 doing the curl.) Guylyn said in the newspaper after finishing in the final ten: "I really appreciated Boyd's help with my training program. It gave me confidence that I had smoothed out any rough spots." Be sure your program is balanced. Include at least one exercise for your bicep in your program.

Procedure An underhand grip is used for the barbell curl. Attempt to decrease unwanted movements, such as rocking back or forward. Concentrate on the muscle as it contracts your fist toward the shoulder. This exercise should be performed slowly and smoothly.

Value This exercise will develop the biceps (front of upper arm). This should serve as a major exercise in your program.

Equipment A regular exercise bar or E-Z curl bar may be used.

Supplementary Exercises for the Bicep

8:5A Preacher barbell curl

8:5B Seated dumbbell curl

8:5C Incline dumbbell curl

Preacher Barbell Curl (8:5A)

Procedure Place the elbows and upper arms on the preacher curl pad so the elbows have just barely locked out. Then, do a slow, controlled curl until the bar is curled up near the chin. This exercise should be performed slowly and smoothly throughout the full range of motion.

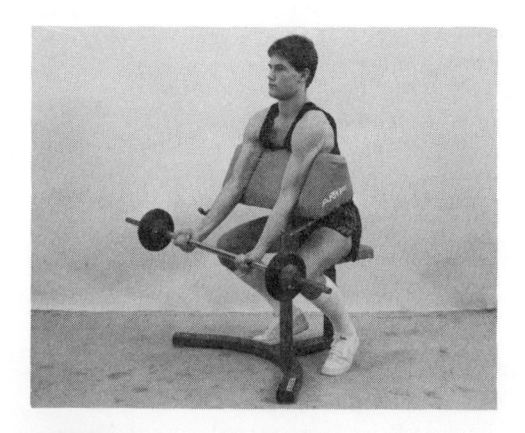

Figure 8.31
Preacher Barbell Curl—Start

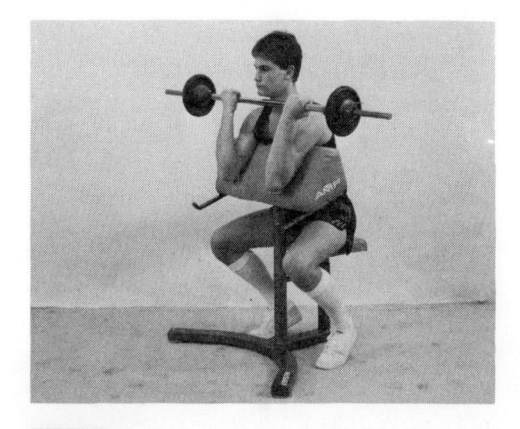

Figure 8.32
Preacher Barbell Curl—Finish

Value This exercise will develop the biceps (front of upper arm). This could serve as a major exercise in place of the barbell curl in your program.

Equipment A preacher curl bench and E-Z curl or barbell are needed.

Seated Dumbbell Curl (8:5B)

Procedure When performing the dumbbell arm curl, use the underhand grip with the arm hanging straight down. After each repetition, straighten the arm all the way. This will put a greater stretch on the muscle. Curl each dumbbell separately while concentrating on each arm. Curl the dumbbell upward until the muscle is fully contracted. The dumbbell arm curl may be performed either standing or sitting down. This exercise should be performed slowly and smoothly.

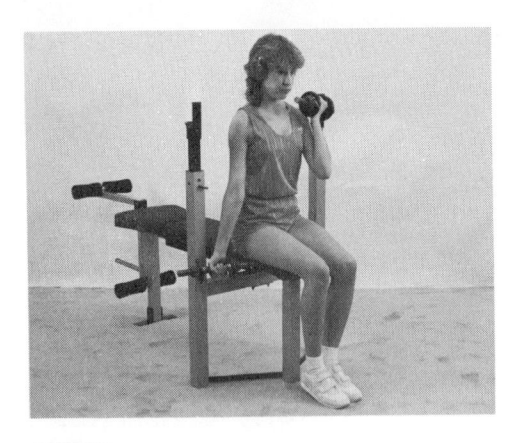

Figure 8.33
Seated Dumbbell Curl—
Start

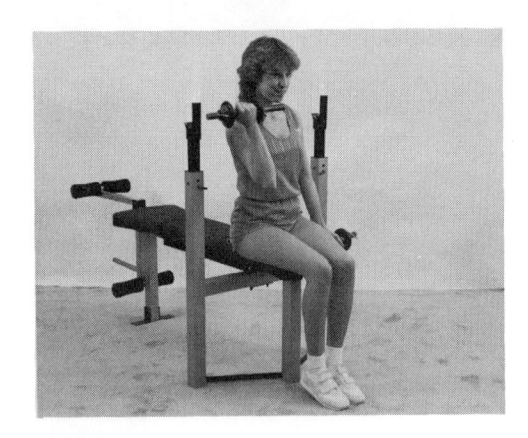

Figure 8.34
Seated Dumbbell Curl—
Finish

Value This exercise will develop the biceps.

Equipment Dumbbells, in addition to a bench or stool, are needed for this exercise.

Incline Dumbbell Curl (8:5C)

Procedure Sit on the incline and lean back. Allow the dumbbells to hang at arm's length with the palms facing forward. Lift the dumbbell with the right hand and let it down, then lift with the left hand. This exercise should be performed slowly and smoothly.

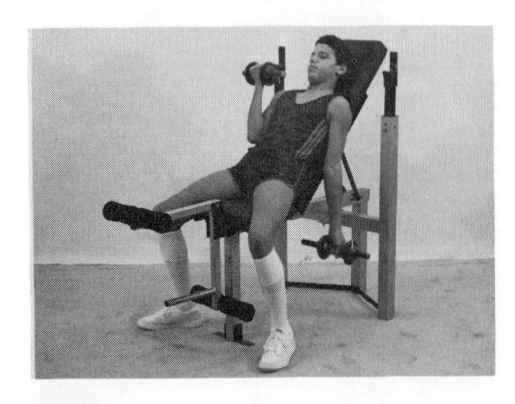

Figure 8.35
Incline Dumbbell Curl—Start

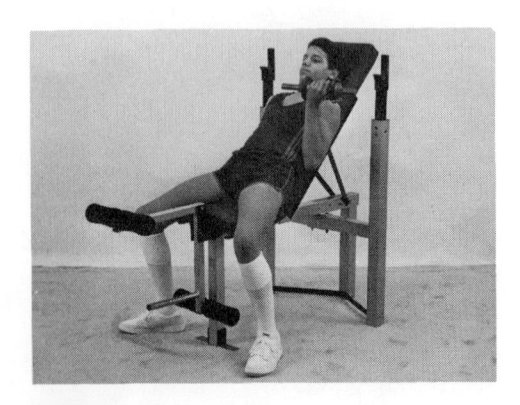

Figure 8.36
Incline Dumbbell Curl—
Finish

Value This exercise will develop the biceps.

Equipment Dumbbells, as well as an incline bench at a 45 degree angle, are required for this exercise.

Tricep Extension (8:6)

This exercise works the large muscle on the back of the upper arm, or the tricep. The tricep is more involved in athletic performance than its counterpart, the bicep—which is on the front side of the upper arm. The development of the tricep is very important to the young athlete. Rich Glover says, "As a middle guard who weighed 210 pounds, I needed additional strength to help me with all aspects of football. Boyd's program helped me gain 24 pounds, and developed my arms, shoulders, and legs, which allowed me to take on the center better." Rich really showed his strength when he went up against an All-American center in the "game of the century." Nebraska's 1971 national championship football team beat number-two-ranked Oklahoma 35–31, in a real shoot-out.

Because of his efforts, Rich Glover finished third in the voting for the Heisman Trophy, which is usually reserved for running backs or quarterbacks. Rich Glover did win the Outland Trophy and the Lombardi Award, in addition to being All-American in 1971 and 1972, and was the UPI Lineman of the Year in 1972. Rich is still considered by many to be the finest middle guard to ever play college football. Rich was not very strong when he started liting, but he gained his strength very quickly. On his tricep extension he improved by fifty pounds in less than three weeks.

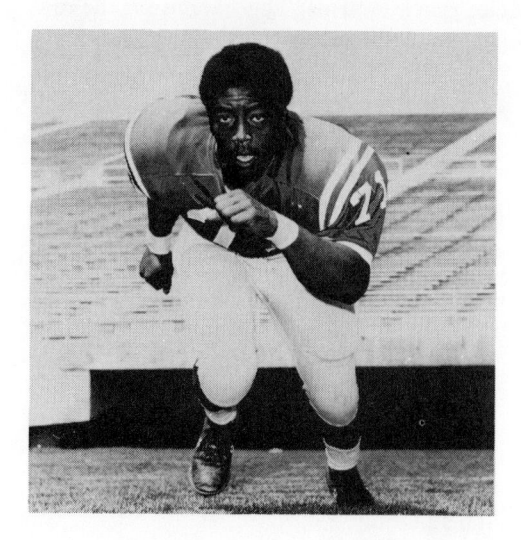

Figure 8.37
Rich Glover was the first player to win both the Outland and Lombardi Awards.

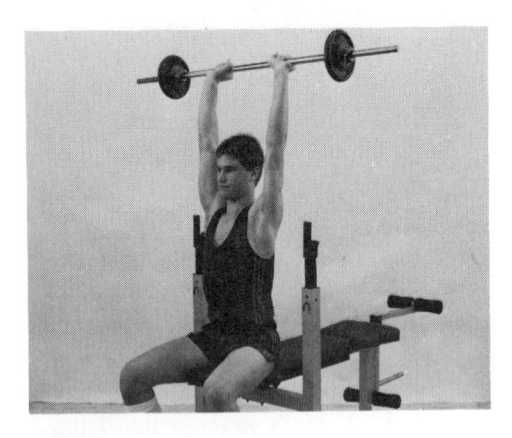

Figure 8.38
Tricep Extension—Start

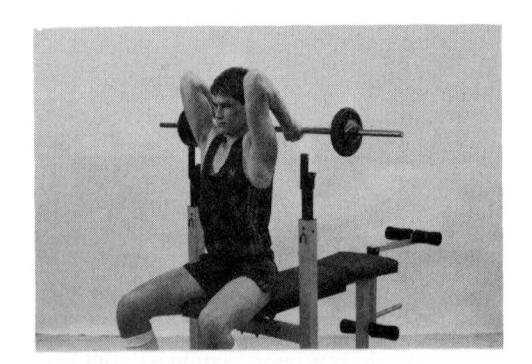

Figure 8.39
Tricep Extension—Finish

Procedure Hold the bar overhead at arm's length, and position the hands about four to six inches apart. Lower the bar downward and backward as you flex the arms at the elbows. The elbows should be kept as high and as far back as possible. Sometimes too much weight is used and the bar is pressed upward. Keep the elbows stationary near the head. This exercise should be performed slowly and smoothly. This exercise can be done seated or standing.

Value This exercise will develop the tricep muscles (back of arm). This exercise is the recommended major exercise for the tricep.

Equipment A barbell, E-Z curl bar, or a dumbbell may be used for this exercise, along with a stool or bench if done seated.

Supplementary Exercises for the Tricep

8:6A Lying tricep extension

8:6B Dips

Lying Tricep Extension (8:6A)

Procedure As you are lying on your back, the hands should be about four to six inches apart. Keep the elbows in the same position, with the upper arm perpendicular to the floor. Raise the bar by extending the arm, keeping the elbows fixed. Lower the bar down past the forehead. This exercise should be performed slowly and smoothly.

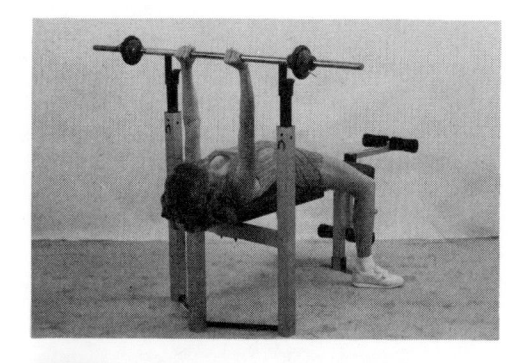

Figure 8.40
Lying Tricep Extension—Start

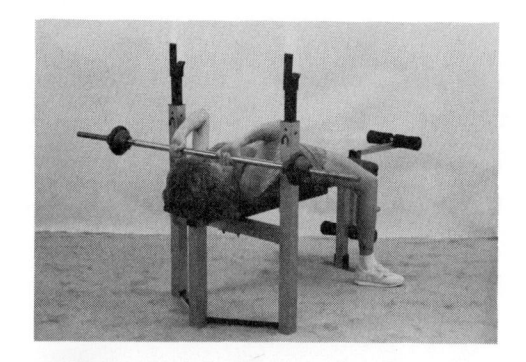

Figure 8.41
Lying Tricep Extension—90 degree position

Value This exercise will develop the tricep muscle (back of arm). This could serve as a major exercise in place of the tricep extension.

Equipment A regular bar, or E–Z curl bar, is needed, in addition to a tricep bench.

Safety Be careful not to drop the bar on your forehead. You may want to have a spotter assist you on this exercise.

Dips (8:6B)

Procedure Support your body weight on the dip bars by locking out the elbows. Lower the body until the upper arm is below horizontal, and then raise the body by extending the arms. For those who lack sufficient strength, a chair may be used to take weight off the arms. Once sufficient strength is reached, the chair will not be needed. For those who have sufficient strength, a weight may be fastened to the waist to increase the intensity of the exercise. This exercise should be performed slowly and smoothly.

Value This exercise will develop the triceps (back of arm), as well as the outer chest muscles and shoulders. This is a supplemental exercise that should require fewer sets than recommended for the major exercises.

Equipment A dip bar station is needed.

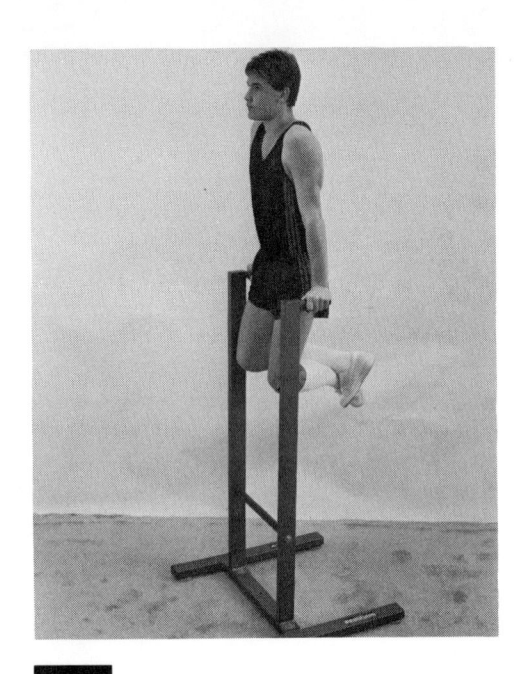

Figure 8.42
Dips—Start

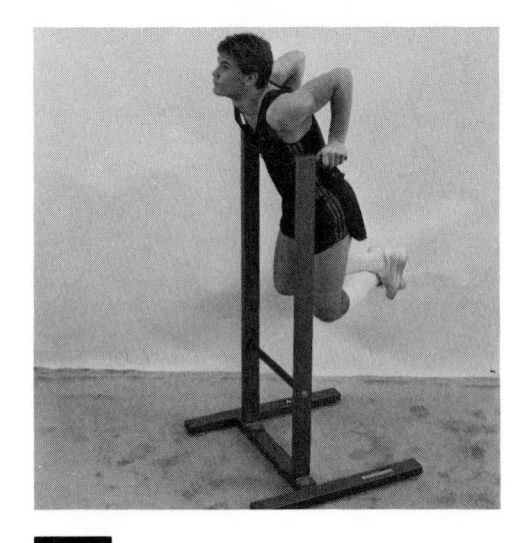

Figure 8.43
Dips—Low Position

CHAPTER NINE

Speed, Power, Agility, and Endurance Drills

Successful athletes are special people who have chosen to excel at a sport, and work very hard to do so. If you really want to become a successful athlete you must have the desire to follow a systematic conditioning program. To become a total athlete, this program must include more than strength development. You'll need to include drills to improve your speed, agility, power, and endurance in conjunction with your lifting routine. This chapter provides you with a six-week schedule to follow. If you are serious about being a successful athlete one day, you must discipline yourself to follow your schedule. If you fail to lift or run when you are supposed to, this means you are not really interested in being the best athlete you can be.

Improve Your Weak Areas

The smart athlete concentrates on improving weak areas. You've probably heard the saying that " a chain is only as strong as its weakest link." A chain is made up of several links. Some of the links are stronger than others. When stress is applied, the weakest link allows the chain to fail. In athletics, your talent is made up of components such as speed, power, agility, and endurance. You will be better in some areas than others. As it was with the chain, any weak area will prevent you from being the best athlete you can be. Find out how you compare to other athletes your age, and then work hard to improve any weak components. To do so you can follow these four steps:

1. Test your speed, power, agility, and endurance.
2. Evaluate your scores.
3. Set goals for improvement.
4. Select drills and follow a program to develop your speed, power, agility, and endurance

Step #1—Testing

You need to test yourself the first day to determine what physical components you'll need to make the most improvement in. Many times athletes think the purpose of conditioning performance tests is to measure or predict future athletic success. This is not the case. Conditioning tests are merely a means of checking various athletic components that contribute to the success of an athlete. Testing points out which athletic components you may have a weakness in and need work on. You may need to have someone help you complete this step. Be sure to write down the date and your performance scores for each test.

Testing for Speed—Fifty-Yard Dash

Equipment and Materials

- One stopwatch (Model #447–315, AMF Hand-Held Watch).
- One person to time.
- One person to start.
- Seventy yards of flat running surface (measure out a fifty-yard course, plus twenty yards for slowing down).

Procedure

1. Stretch and warm-up completely, then take a practice run.
2. When ready, place hand on starting line.
3. Starter gives commands, "Ready?" and "Go."
4. On the command, "Go," starter gives downward sweep of arm as a visual signal for the starter to start stopwatch.
5. Watch is stopped at the moment the runner crosses the finish line.
6. Record three trials to the nearest tenth of a second, and average them. To reduce any possibility of human error, use your average time for the evaluation.

Testing for Power—Standing Long Jump

Equipment and Materials

- A mat or carpeted floor for soft landing surface.
- At least ten feet of jumping area free of obstacles.
- A tape measure at least ten feet long.
- One person to measure your jump (see fig. 9.9 for an illustration of the long jump).

Procedure

1. Allow three trials.
2. Measure from the take-off line to the heel upon landing.
3. Record the best of three trials to the nearest inch.

Testing for Agility—Shuttle Run (Total of 120 Feet)

Equipment and Materials

- Two blocks of wood 2" × 2" × 4".
- Two parallel lines marked thirty feet apart.
- One person to time (fig. 9.11).

Procedure

1. Stretch and warm up, including a practice run.
2. Place blocks of wood behind one of the lines.
3. Start at other line on the commands "Ready?" and "Go."
4. Run to the blocks, pick up one and run back to starting line. Place block behind starting line.
5. Run back and pick up second block, then run back across starting line carrying the block.
6. Allow two trials with adequate rest in between.
7. Record the best time to nearest tenth of a second.

Testing for Endurance—Six Hundred-Yard Run-Walk

Equipment and Materials

- A standard 440-yard track, or area marked to measure six hundred yards in length.
- One person to keep your time.
- A stopwatch.

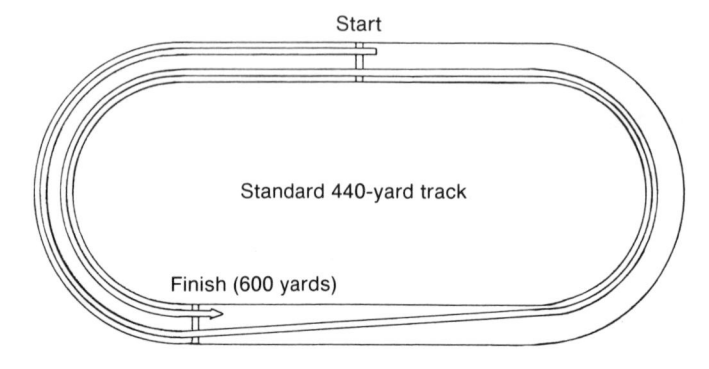

Figure 9.1
Standard 440-Yard Track

Procedure

1. From a standing start, on the commands "Ready?" and "Go", start running the six hundred-yard course.
2. You may walk, if necessary.
3. Record your time in minutes and seconds.

Step Two—Evaluation

After you have been tested, you will want to evaluate how you compare to other boys and girls your age across the nation. You can make this comparison by determining your percentile ranking for your age. This should clearly show you where you need the most improvement. Look over the example profile in table 9.1 to familiarize yourself with the evaluation process.

Table 9.1
Sample Conditioning Profile for Girls—13 Years Old

Percentile	50-Yard Dash	Standing Long Jump	Shuttle Run	600-Yard Run
100th	6.0	8' 0"	7.0	1:43
95th	6.9	6' 5"	9.9	2:04
90th	7.0	6' 2"	10.0	2:12
85th	7.2	6' 0"	10.2	2:16
80th	7.3	5'10"	10.4	2:20
75th	7.4	5' 9"	10.5	2:23
70th	7.5	5' 7"	10.6	2:27
65th	7.6	5' 6"	10.8	2:30
60th	7.7	5' 5"	11.0	2:34
55th	7.9	5' 4"	11.1	2:37
50th	8.0	5' 3"	11.2	2:41
45th	8.0	5' 2"	11.3	2:45
40th	8.1	5' 1"	11.5	2:49
35th	8.2	5' 0"	11.6	2:55
30th	8.3	4'10"	11.9	2:59
25th	8.5	4' 9"	12.0	3:06
20th	8.7	4' 8"	12.2	3:12
15th	8.9	4' 6"	12.6	3:20
10th	9.2	4' 3"	12.8	3:30
5th	10.0	4' 0"	13.2	3:49
0	14.2	3' 2"	16.5	5:10

For example, if you are a 13-year old girl and ran fifty yards in 8.5 seconds, you would refer to table 9.1 to see that you rank in the 25th percentile. This means that, in comparison with other girls 13-years old, 25 percent of the girls are slower and 75 percent are faster. In the other categories your results are in the 50th to 55th percentile. This would mean your weakness is speed, so more emphasis should be placed on speed development, while you continue to work on power, agility, and endurance.

You should now turn to tables 9.3 to 9.8 and fill in on the profile your current testing results for your gender and age. By completing your conditioning profile you will see very quickly what your strengths and weaknesses are. These statistics are provided by the American Alliance of Health, Physical Education, and Recreation.

Step Three—Goal Setting

The establishment of goals is an essential part of your program. Setting goals will convert your desires to become a better athlete into a plan of action. You need something to motivate you in order to become the very best that you can.

Table 9.2
Conditioning Profile for Girls—13 Years Old (Goal Setting)

Percentile	50-Yard Dash	Standing Long Jump	Shuttle Run	600-Yard Run
100th	6.0	8' 0"	7.0	1:43
95th	6.9	6' 5"	9.9	2:04
90th	7.0	6' 2"	10.0	2:12
85th	7.2	6' 0"	10.2	2:16
80th	7.3	5'10"	10.4	2:20
75th	7.4	5' 9"	10.5	2:23
70th	7.5	5' 7"	10.6	2:27
65th	7.6	5' 6"	10.8	2:30
60th	7.7	5' 5"	11.0	2:34
55th	7.9	5' 4"	11.1	2:37
50th	8.0	5' 3"	11.2	2:41
45th	8.0	5' 2"	11.3	2:45
40th	8.1	5' 1"	11.5	2:49
35th	8.2	5' 0"	11.6	2:55
30th	8.3	4'10"	11.9	2:59
25th	8.5	4' 9"	12.0	3:06
20th	8.7	4' 8"	12.2	3:12
15th	8.9	4' 6"	12.6	3:20
10th	9.2	4' 3"	12.8	3:30
5th	10.0	4' 0"	13.2	3:49
0	14.2	3' 2"	16.5	5:10

Before setting your own goals, study table 9.2. For example, if you were a 13-year old girl, your present levels would be represented by the solid line. The dotted line would represent your goals, or where you would like to be at the end of your present program. Notice the goals are demanding, yet realistic. Make sure you don't set your personal goals so high that you don't think you can actually reach them.

Simply decide what level of conditioning you can feasibly reach, then circle that level on the conditioning profile for your gender and age on tables 9.3 to 9.8. This goal setting process will not be effective unless you have the desire to work hard enough to overcome any obstacles that might be in your path, preventing you from reaching your goals.

Table 9.3a
Conditioning Profile for Boys—12 Years Old

Percentile	50-Yard Dash	Standing Long Jump	Shuttle Run	600-Yard Run
100th	6.3	7' 5"	6.8	1:38
95th	6.8	6' 6"	9.6	1:52
90th	7.0	6' 3"	9.8	1:57
85th	7.1	6' 1"	10.0	2:00
80th	7.3	6' 0"	10.0	2:04
75th	7.4	5'11"	10.2	2:06
70th	7.5	5' 9"	10.3	2:09
65th	7.5	5' 8"	10.4	2:11
60th	7.6	5' 7"	10.5	2:14
55th	7.7	5' 6"	10.6	2:16
50th	7.8	5' 5"	10.7	2:19
45th	7.9	5' 4"	10.8	2:22
40th	8.0	5' 3"	11.0	2:24
35th	8.1	5' 2"	11.1	2:28
30th	8.2	5' 1"	11.3	2:32
25th	8.3	5' 0"	11.4	2:37
20th	8.5	4'10"	11.6	2:42
15th	8.6	4' 9"	11.8	2:48
10th	9.0	4' 6"	12.0	2:54
5th	9.5	4' 2"	12.4	3:06
0	11.3	3' 2"	22.0	4:10

Table 9.3b
Conditioning Profile for Girls—12 Years Old

Percentile	50-Yard Dash	Standing Long Jump	Shuttle Run	600-Yard Run
100th	6.0	7' 0"	8.5	1:40
95th	7.0	6' 2"	9.9	2:06
90th	7.2	6' 0"	10.2	2:14
85th	7.4	5' 9"	10.5	2:21
80th	7.5	5' 8"	10.6	2:23
75th	7.6	5' 6"	10.8	2:26
70th	7.7	5' 5"	10.9	2:31
65th	7.9	5' 4"	11.0	2:35
60th	8.0	5' 2"	11.1	2:39
55th	8.0	5' 1"	11.2	2:43
50th	8.1	5' 0"	11.4	2:47
45th	8.2	4'11"	11.5	2:51
40th	8.3	4'10"	11.5	2:56
35th	8.4	4' 9"	11.7	3:00
30th	8.5	4' 8"	11.8	3:06
25th	8.7	4' 6"	12.0	3:13
20th	8.9	4' 5"	12.1	3:19
15th	9.1	4' 3"	12.5	3:27
10th	9.4	4' 2"	13.0	3:36
5th	10.0	3'10"	13.3	3:59
0	14.9	3'00"	15.3	6:02

Table 9.4a
Conditioning Profile for Boys—13 Years Old

Percentile	50-Yard Dash	Standing Long Jump	Shuttle Run	600-Yard Run
100th	5.8	8' 6"	7.0	1:26
95th	6.5	7' 1"	9.3	1:45
90th	6.7	6'10"	9.5	1:50
85th	6.9	6' 8"	9.7	1:54
80th	7.0	6' 5"	9.8	1:57
75th	7.0	6' 3"	10.0	1:59
70th	7.1	6' 2"	10.0	2:01
65th	7.2	6' 0"	10.1	2:03
60th	7.3	6' 0"	10.2	2:05
55th	7.4	5'10"	10.3	2:07
50th	7.5	5' 9"	10.4	2:10
45th	7.5	5' 7"	10.5	2:13
40th	7.6	5' 6"	10.6	2:15
35th	7.7	5' 5"	10.8	2:20
30th	7.9	5' 3"	11.0	2:24
25th	8.0	5' 2"	11.0	2:27
20th	8.1	5' 0"	11.3	2:32
15th	8.3	4'10"	11.5	2:37
10th	8.7	4' 7"	11.8	2:45
5th	9.0	4' 4"	12.4	3:00
0	15.0	3' 3"	16.0	4:00

Table 9.4b
Conditioning Profile for Girls—13 Years Old

Percentile	50-Yard Dash	Standing Long Jump	Shuttle Run	600-Yard Run
100th	6.0	8' 0"	7.0	1:43
95th	6.9	6' 5"	9.9	2:04
90th	7.0	6' 2"	10.0	2:12
85th	7.2	6' 0"	10.2	2:16
80th	7.3	5'10"	10.4	2:20
75th	7.4	5' 9"	10.5	2:23
70th	7.5	5' 7"	10.6	2:27
65th	7.6	5' 6"	10.8	2:30
60th	7.7	5' 5"	11.0	2:34
55th	7.9	5' 4"	11.0	2:37
50th	8.0	5' 3"	11.2	2:41
45th	8.0	5' 2"	11.3	2:45
40th	8.1	5' 1"	11.5	2:49
35th	8.2	5' 0"	11.6	2:55
30th	8.3	4'10"	11.9	2:59
25th	8.5	4' 9"	12.0	3:06
20th	8.7	4' 8"	12.2	3:12
15th	8.9	4' 6"	12.6	3:20
10th	9.2	4' 3"	12.8	3:30
5th	10.0	4' 0"	13.2	3:49
0	14.2	3' 2"	16.5	5:10

Table 9.5a
Conditioning Profile for Boys—14 Years Old

Percentile	50-Yard Dash	Standing Long Jump	Shuttle Run	600-Yard Run
100th	5.9	9' 0"	7.0	1:27
95th	6.2	7' 6"	8.9	1:39
90th	6.4	7' 2"	9.2	1:44
85th	6.5	6'11"	9.3	1:47
80th	6.6	6'10"	9.5	1:50
75th	6.8	6' 8"	9.6	1:52
70th	6.9	6' 6"	9.8	1:55
65th	7.0	6' 6"	9.8	1:57
60th	7.0	6' 4"	10.0	1:58
55th	7.1	6' 3"	10.0	2:00
50th	7.2	6' 2"	10.1	2:03
45th	7.3	6' 1"	10.1	2:05
40th	7.4	5'11"	10.2	2:07
35th	7.5	5'10"	10.4	2:10
30th	7.6	5' 8"	10.6	2:12
25th	7.7	5' 6"	10.7	2:16
20th	7.9	5' 4"	10.9	2:22
15th	8.0	5' 2"	11.0	2:30
10th	8.2	5' 0"	11.3	2:37
5th	8.8	4' 8"	11.9	2:51
0	11.1	2' 0"	18.6	6:00

Table 9.5b
Conditioning Profile for Girls—14 Years Old

Percentile	50-Yard Dash	Standing Long Jump	Shuttle Run	600-Yard Run
100th	6.0	7' 5"	7.8	1:33
95th	6.8	6' 8"	9.7	2:02
90th	7.0	6' 5"	10.0	2:07
85th	7.1	6' 3"	10.1	2:11
80th	7.2	6' 0"	10.2	2:15
75th	7.3	5'11"	10.3	2:19
70th	7.4	5'10"	10.5	2:24
65th	7.5	5' 8"	10.6	2:29
60th	7.6	5' 7"	10.7	2:32
55th	7.6	5' 6"	10.9	2:36
50th	7.8	5' 4"	11.0	2:40
45th	7.9	5' 3"	11.2	2:44
40th	8.0	5' 2"	11.4	2:47
35th	8.0	5' 1"	11.5	2:51
30th	8.2	4'11"	11.7	2:56
25th	8.3	4'10"	12.0	3:01
20th	8.5	4' 9"	12.1	3:08
15th	8.8	4' 6"	12.3	3:16
10th	9.0	4' 4"	12.8	3:27
5th	9.6	4' 0"	13.1	3:49
0	11.0	3' 0"	19.2	5:00

Table 9.6a
Conditioning Profile for Boys—15 Years Old

Percentile	50-Yard Dash	Standing Long Jump	Shuttle Run	600-Yard Run
100th	5.5	9' 0''	7.0	1:20
95th	6.0	8' 0''	8.9	1:36
90th	6.2	7' 7''	9.1	1:40
85th	6.3	7' 5''	9.2	1:42
80th	6.4	7' 3''	9.3	1:45
75th	6.5	7' 2''	9.4	1:46
70th	6.6	7' 0''	9.5	1:48
65th	6.6	6'11''	9.6	1:50
60th	6.8	6'10''	9.7	1:52
55th	6.8	6' 9''	9.8	1:54
50th	6.9	6' 8''	9.9	1:56
45th	6.9	6' 6''	10.0	1:57
40th	7.0	6' 5''	10.0	1:59
35th	7.1	6' 4''	10.1	2:01
30th	7.2	6' 3''	10.2	2:05
25th	7.3	6' 1''	10.4	2:08
20th	7.4	5'11''	10.5	2:11
15th	7.5	5' 9''	10.8	2:15
10th	7.6	5' 6''	11.1	2:23
5th	8.0	5' 2''	11.7	2:30
0	11.0	2' 0''	14.7	4:39

Table 9.6b
Conditioning Profile for Girls—15 Years Old

Percentile	50-Yard Dash	Standing Long Jump	Shuttle Run	600-Yard Run
100th	6.0	8' 0''	7.4	1:41
95th	6.9	6' 7''	9.9	2:00
90th	7.0	6' 3''	10.0	2:10
85th	7.1	6' 1''	10.2	2:14
80th	7.2	6' 0''	10.3	2:18
75th	7.4	5'10''	10.4	2:22
70th	7.5	5' 9''	10.5	2:25
65th	7.5	5' 8''	10.6	2:28
60th	7.6	5' 6''	10.9	2:30
55th	7.7	5' 6''	11.0	2:34
50th	7.8	5' 5''	11.0	2:37
45th	7.9	5' 3''	11.1	2:40
40th	8.0	5' 2''	11.3	2:45
35th	8.0	5' 1''	11.4	2:50
30th	8.1	5' 0''	11.6	2:55
25th	8.2	4'11''	11.8	3:00
20th	8.4	4' 9''	12.0	3:05
15th	8.6	4' 7''	12.2	3:12
10th	8.8	4' 5''	12.6	3:26
5th	9.2	4' 2''	13.3	3:28
0	15.6	3' 0''	18.5	5:58

Table 9.7a
Conditioning Profile for Boys—16 Years Old

Percentile	50-Yard Dash	Standing Long Jump	Shuttle Run	600-Yard Run
100th	5.5	9' 2''	7.3	1:21
95th	6.0	8' 2''	8.6	1:34
90th	6.2	7'11''	8.9	1:38
85th	6.3	7' 9''	9.1	1:40
80th	6.4	7' 6''	9.2	1:42
75th	6.5	7' 6''	9.3	1:44
70th	6.5	7' 4''	9.4	1:46
65th	6.6	7' 3''	9.5	1:48
60th	6.6	7' 2''	9.6	1:49
55th	6.7	7' 1''	9.7	1:50
50th	6.7	7' 0''	9.9	1:52
45th	6.8	6'11''	10.0	1:54
40th	6.8	6' 9''	10.0	1:56
35th	6.9	6' 8''	10.1	1:58
30th	7.0	6' 7''	10.3	1:59
25th	7.0	6' 6''	10.5	2:01
20th	7.1	6' 4''	10.6	2:04
15th	7.2	6' 2''	10.9	2:09
10th	7.4	5'11''	11.1	2:17
5th	7.7	5' 5''	11.9	2:31
0	9.9	3' 4''	15.0	4:11

Table 9.7b
Conditioning Profile for Girls—16 Years Old

Percentile	50-Yard Dash	Standing Long Jump	Shuttle Run	600-Yard Run
100th	5.6	7' 7''	7.8	1:45
95th	7.0	6' 6''	10.0	2:08
90th	7.1	6' 3''	10.2	2:15
85th	7.3	6' 0''	10.4	2:19
80th	7.4	5'11''	10.5	2:21
75th	7.5	5' 9''	10.6	2:26
70th	7.5	5' 8''	10.8	2:29
65th	7.6	5' 6''	10.9	2:32
60th	7.7	5' 6''	11.0	2:36
55th	7.8	5' 4''	11.1	2:39
50th	7.9	5' 3''	11.2	2:43
45th	8.0	5' 2''	11.4	2:47
40th	8.0	5' 1''	11.5	2:49
35th	8.1	5' 0''	11.7	2:54
30th	8.2	4'10''	11.9	2:58
25th	8.3	4' 9''	12.0	3:03
20th	8.5	4' 7''	12.1	3:09
15th	8.5	4' 6''	12.5	3:18
10th	8.8	4' 4''	12.8	3:30
5th	9.3	4' 0''	13.7	3:49
0	15.6	2' 8''	24.9	5:05

Table 9.8a
Conditioning Profile for Boys—17 Years Old

Percentile	50-Yard Dash	Standing Long Jump	Shuttle Run	600-Yard Run
100th	5.4	9'10"	8.0	1:20
95th	5.9	8' 5"	8.6	1:32
90th	6.0	8' 2"	8.9	1:35
85th	6.1	8' 0"	9.0	1:38
80th	6.3	7'10"	9.1	1:41
75th	6.3	7' 9"	9.2	1:43
70th	6.4	7' 7"	9.3	1:45
65th	6.5	7' 6"	9.4	1:47
60th	6.5	7' 6"	9.5	1:49
55th	6.6	7' 3"	9.6	1:50
50th	6.6	7' 2"	9.8	1:52
45th	6.7	7' 1"	9.9	1:53
40th	6.8	7' 0"	10.0	1:56
35th	6.9	6'10"	10.1	1:57
30th	7.0	6' 8"	10.2	1:59
25th	7.0	6' 6"	10.4	2:02
20th	7.1	6' 4"	10.5	2:06
15th	7.3	6' 2"	10.7	2:12
10th	7.5	5'10"	11.0	2:22
5th	7.9	5' 3"	11.7	2:38
0	12.0	3' 0"	15.7	5:10

Table 9.8b
Conditioning Profile for Girls—17 Years Old

Percentile	50-Yard Dash	Standing Long Jump	Shuttle Run	600-Yard Run
100th	6.4	7' 6"	8.2	1:39
95th	6.8	6' 9"	9.6	2:02
90th	7.0	6' 6"	10.0	2:10
85th	7.1	6' 3"	10.1	2:14
80th	7.3	6' 2"	10.3	2:20
75th	7.4	6' 0"	10.4	2:24
70th	7.5	5'11"	10.5	2:26
65th	7.5	5'10"	10.7	2:30
60th	7.6	5' 9"	10.9	2:35
55th	7.7	5' 7"	11.0	2:38
50th	7.9	5' 5"	11.1	2:41
45th	8.0	5' 4"	11.3	2:45
40th	8.0	5' 3"	11.5	2:48
35th	8.1	5' 2"	11.6	2:53
30th	8.2	5' 0"	11.9	2:56
25th	8.4	4'11"	12.0	3:02
20th	8.5	4' 9"	12.2	3:09
15th	8.8	4' 7"	12.5	3:19
10th	9.0	4' 4"	13.0	3:30
5th	9.5	4' 1"	14.0	3:45
0	15.0	3' 3"	17.0	6:40

Step Four—Your Program

After you have tested, evaluated your scores, and set goals for improvement, it is time to begin a program to develop your speed, power, agility, and endurance.

Speed

Speed is simply the product of stride length and stride frequency. Stride length is the distance that you cover with each step as you run. Stride frequency is the number of steps that you take per second. Your speed can be improved by increasing your stride length and/or stride frequency.

You cannot reach your full speed potential by simply running sprints. A number of training elements must be fused together in order to achieve maximum speed potential. Speed is often hindered by mechanically poor running form. Stride length and stride frequency can be greatly enhanced by working on the speed drills that improve technique. This helps you to develop a mechanically efficient sprint form.

Most experts on speed training tend to agree that the best results are attained by concentrating your efforts on improving stride length. Improvement of stride length is best accomplished by increasing the forces produced by the muscular contraction of the leg and hip muscles against the ground. Strength training and the power drills in the next section enable you to contract your muscles more forcefully. Strength training, plyometrics, and flexibility drills to improve technique, must be combined with running sprints into an effective program to develop maximum speed.

Speed Drills

Drill #1 High Knees

Value Develops the muscles for a fast, long stride, and adds flexibility in the hamstrings.

Procedure

1. Drive knees high and forcefully.
2. When one leg is lifted, the other leg should be fully extended.
3. Bend forward slightly at the waist; keep back straight.
4. Drill can be done with or without arms.
5. When arms are used, drive elbows back and up vigorously.
6. Relax face and arms.
7. Take short, quick, one-foot steps.

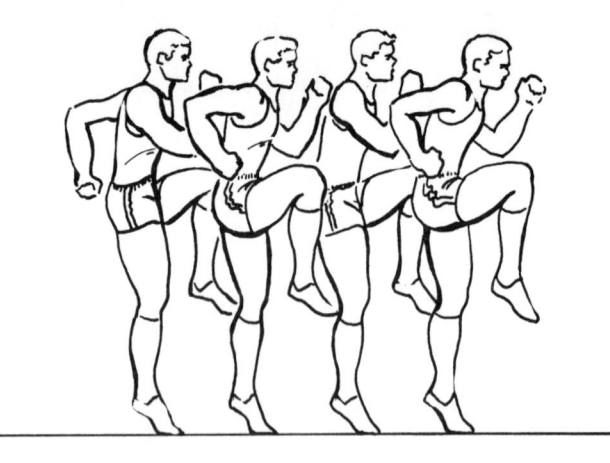

Figure 9.2
High Knees

Avoid

- Low knee lift.
- Incomplete extension of the legs fully at ankle, knee, and hip joints.
- Leaning back.
- Taking steps longer than one foot.
- Tensing face and arms

Drill #2 Heel Ups

Value Develops strength in the hamstring, and active flexibility in quadriceps.

Procedure

1. Alternately swing heel of each foot up to buttocks.
2. Be sure action is quick; smooth swinging motion produced largely at knee joint.

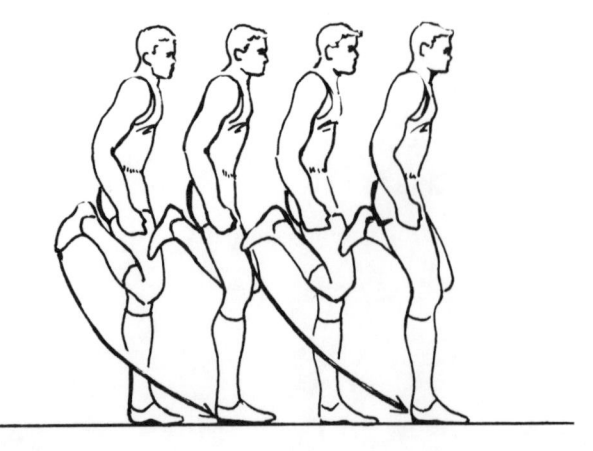

Figure 9.3
Heel-Ups

Avoid

- Moving forward too fast.
- Using arms.
- Lifting the knees by flexing at the hips.

Drill #3 Ankle Flips

Value To develop explosive strength in calf muscles.

Procedure

1. Alternately explode from foot to foot as high as possible using only the ankle action.
2. Land high on the toes and settle down to the heel.
3. Keep knees and hips rigid.
4. Keep arms relaxed at the sides.

Avoid

- Achieving too much distance on each explosion.
- Flexing knees and hips.
- Swinging feet out to the side.
- Using arms.

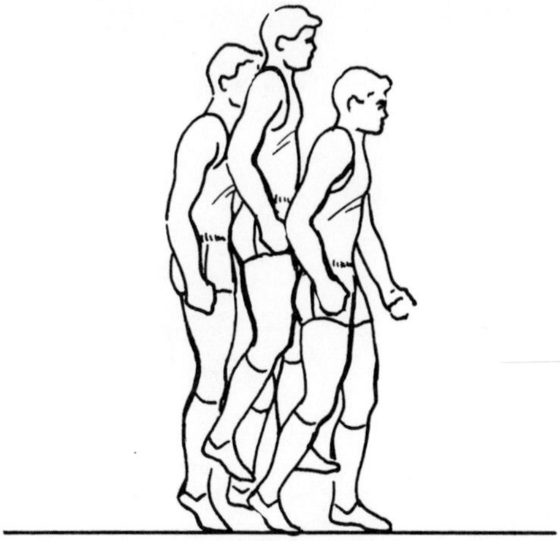

Figure 9.4
Ankle Flips

Drill #4 Form Starts

Value Improvement of stance.

Procedure

1. Front foot is placed three to six inches behind starting line.
2. The hand opposite the front foot should be high with fingertips directly on the starting line, with thumb and forefinger parallel to the line.
3. The other hand is placed on the hip of the forward leg, with elbow pointed up.
4. The back foot is six to twelve inches behind the heel of the forward foot, and two to four inches to the side.
5. The hips should be slightly above shoulder height.
6. Shoulders should be slightly in front of the starting line, with the majority of the body weight on the front leg and hand.
7. Eyes focused two to three feet in front of the starting line.

Avoid

- Placing front foot back too far.
- Placing hands on knuckles of fingers.
- Resting arm on front leg.
- Keeping the hips lower than the shoulders.
- Placing the weight on back leg.
- Holding head up.

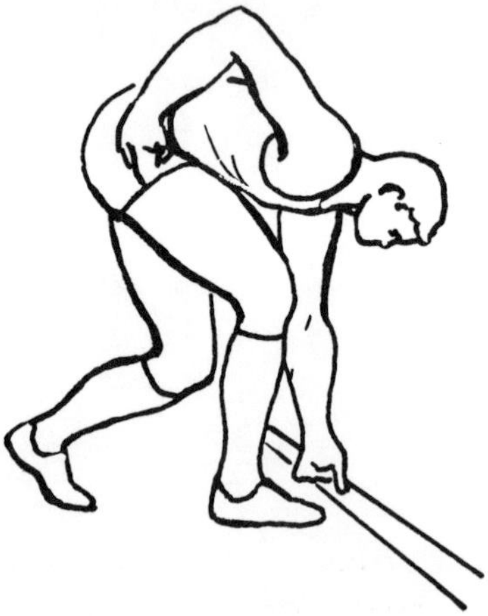

Figure 9.5
Form Starts

Drill #5 Form Starts

Value Improvement of start.

Procedure

1. Pull back leg forcefully forward with a quick and long first step.
2. Straighten front leg explosively, by extending at ankle, knee, and hip.
3. Bring elbow of support arm forcefully up and back.
4. Drive hand on the hip straight forward.
5. Move hips forward.
6. Keep head down.
7. Relax neck, face, jaw, and hands.

Avoid

- Standing straight up coming out of the blocks.
- Looking up by lifting the head.
- Using the front leg for the first step.
- Not extending front leg completely at ankle, knee, and hip.
- Driving arms across the body.
- Twisting feet to side when driving out.
- Tension in neck, face, jaws, and hands.

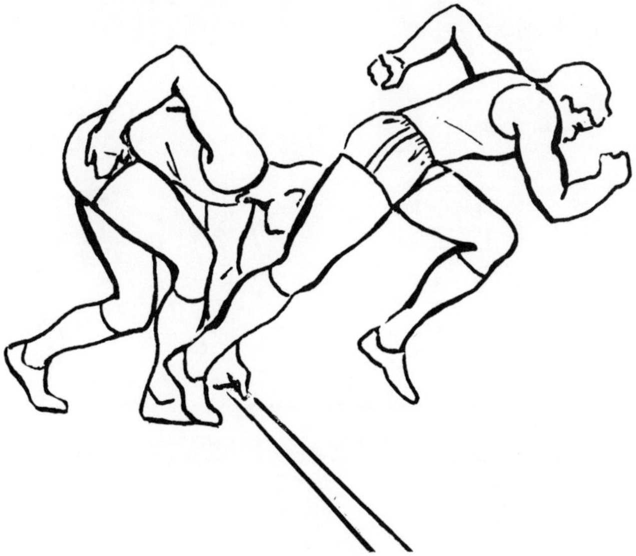

Figure 9.6
Form Starts

Drill # 6 Form Sprints

Value To develop proper sprinting technique.

Procedure Concentrate on the Following Points

1. Drive off back leg, extending completely at ankles, knees, and hips.
2. Swing heel up to the hip.
3. Carry leg to high knee, so thigh is parallel with the ground.
4. Reach with the front leg.
5. Arms at a 90 degree angle, swinging independently of the shoulders, straight forward and back.
6. On the backswing, drive elbows back and up.
7. On forward swing, bring hand to level of the shoulders.
8. Focus eyes twenty to thirty yards ahead.
9. Relax hands, shoulders, neck, and face.

Avoid

- Incomplete extension of legs.
- Turning toes outward.
- Heel not coming up to hips.
- Thigh not coming through to a parallel position with ground.
- Not reaching with the front leg.
- Not driving elbow back.
- Raising hand above shoulders on forward swing.
- Driving arms across the body.
- Excessive head movement.
- Tension in hands, shoulders, neck, and face.

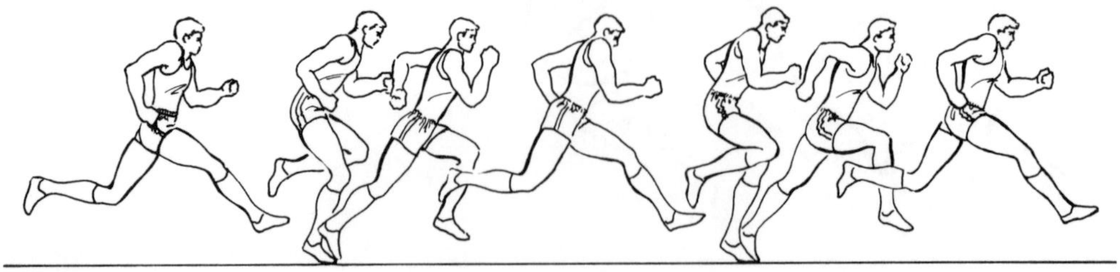

Figure 9.7
Form Sprints

Power

Power is the combination of strength and speed. It refers to an athlete's ability to apply maximum force in the shortest period of time possible. It is essential in such sports as football (blocking and tackling), baseball (throwing and hitting), and basketball (jumping). Your power will increase as you increase your speed and/or strength.

Power can be greatly enhanced by simply doing the squat, hip sled, or lunge. Your strength training should be supplemented by drills called *plyometrics*. Plyometrics cause your muscles to contract forcibly and quickly.

Power (Plyometric) Drills

Drill #1 Bounding

Value To increase stride length.

Procedure

1. Explode forward from one leg to the other, achieving maximum distance on each stride.
2. Drive off the balls of the feet.
3. Bring the thighs parallel with the ground.
4. Pump the arms vigorously in coordination with leg movements.
5. Make your movements exaggerated, with explosive, flowing, harmonious action.
6. Move at one-fourth to one-third of your running speed.
7. Relax.

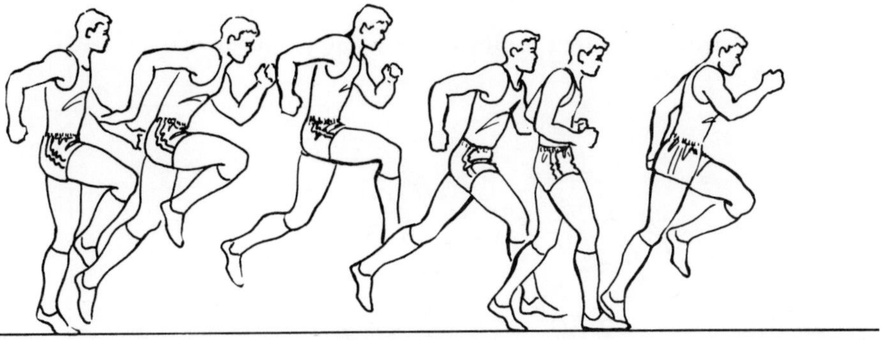

Figure 9.8
Bounding

Avoid

- Achieving too much height.
- Going too fast.
- Tension in hands, neck, and face.

Drill #2 Long Jump

Value Develops explosiveness for starting power and acceleration.

Procedure

1. Stand with feet parallel and hip-width apart, with toes pointed straight ahead.
2. Swing arms backward and bend at the knees and hips.
3. Explosively jump up and forward (45 degree angle) by simultaneously swinging the arms forward and extending the legs.
4. While in the air, pull the knees up to the body.
5. Land by extending the legs forward.
6. Jump for as much distance as possible.

Avoid

- Spacing feet too wide apart.
- Turning the toes outward just prior to jump.
- Bending too much at knees and hips.
- Jumping without the use of arms.
- Incompletely extending legs at ankle, knee, and hip joints.
- Jumping too high or low.
- Keeping legs straight while in flight.

Note: The following drills are variations of the long jump (fig. 9.9).

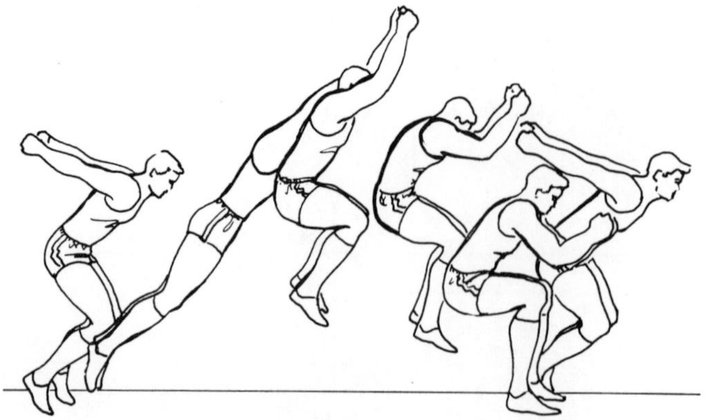

Figure 9.9 Long Jumps

Drill #3A Power Jumping

Jump as far as possible for three to seven jumps.

Drill #3B Speed Jumping

Jump as fast as possible for distance of twenty to forty yards.

Drill #4 Single Leg Hop

Value To develop explosiveness for starting power and acceleration.

Procedure

1. Stand balanced on one foot, with toes pointed straight ahead.
2. Swing arms backward and bend leg at knee and hip.
3. Explosively hop forward and up (45 degree angle) by simultaneously swinging arms forward and extending the legs.
4. Lift the knee high as you take off.
5. Go for as much distance as possible.
6. Land on both feet.

Avoid

- Turning toes outward just prior to the hop.
- Incompletely extending legs at ankle, knee, and hip joints.
- Hopping too high or low.

Note: The following drills are variations of the single leg hop. You need to learn the procedure for the single leg hop (fig. 9.10) so that you can incorporate it into the hopping drills.

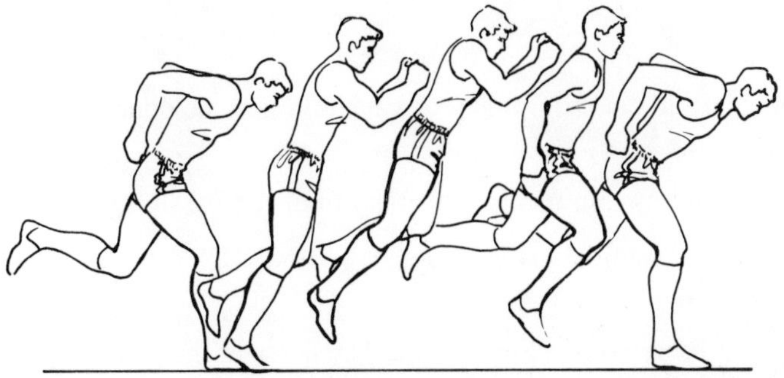

Figure 9.10
Single Leg Hops

Drill #5A 10/10 Hopping

Starting on the right leg, hop as fast as possible for ten yards. Switch immediately to the left leg and hop another ten yards. Alternate from right to left for a total of forty to sixty yards. Emphasize hopping as fast as possible.

Drill #5B Power Hopping

On one leg, hop for as much distance as possible for three to seven hops. Repeat using the other leg.

Agility

Agility refers to an athlete's ability to change directions rapidly, while maintaining balance without the loss of speed. An athlete must have good agility to be successful in activities such as football, baseball, basketball, volleyball, or racquetball.

Your agility can be greatly enhanced by developing additional strength, speed, and power, but these components must be synchronized in a smooth, flowing motion. It would be wise to include agility drills when setting up your training program. The drills should incorporate forward, lateral, and backward movements. They should also require you to change directions quickly while the body is in awkward positions. Three agility drills are provided here for your consideration, however, you should test, evaluate, and set goals before concentrating on your program.

Agility Drills

Drill #1 Shuttle Run

In addition to being a good test of agility for young athletes, the shuttle (described earlier in this chapter) can also be included as an agility drill.

Drill #2 Nebraska Agility Drill

Value Improvement in agility.

Procedure

1. Place your hand at starting line "A" (fig. 9.12). A variation may be done by lying on your back with head in line "A".
2. On the command of "Go," get up and run forward as rapidly as possible.
3. Make a righthand turn around a milk carton or object on line "B". You may place your right hand on the ground for balance.
4. Run back to the second milk carton on line "A", and make a lefthand turn. You can place your left hand on the ground for balance.
5. Then sprint forward, touch line "B" with your hand, and backpeddle to the finish at line "A".

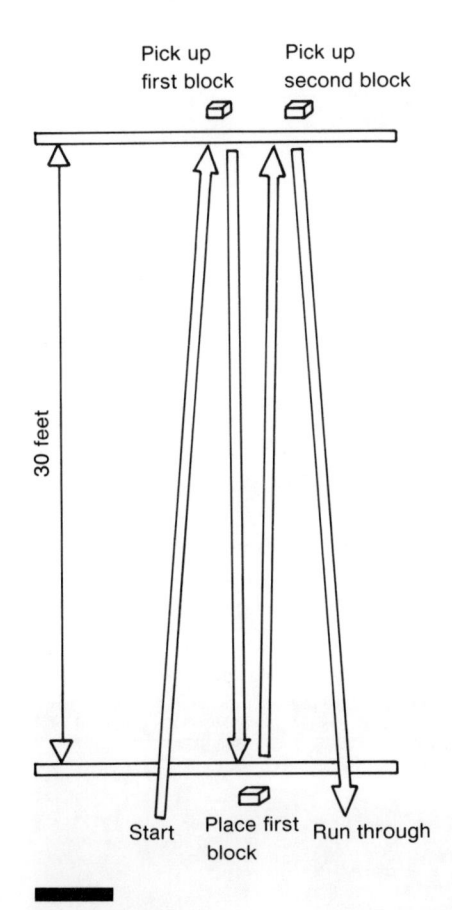

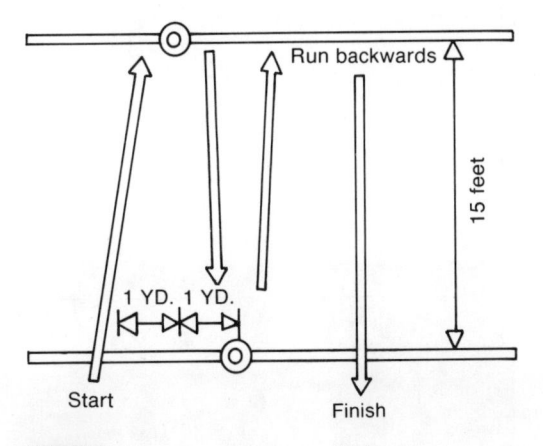

Figure 9.11
Shuttle Run

Figure 9.12
Nebraska Agility Run

Drill #3 Pro Agility Drill

Value Improvement in agility.

Procedure

1. Stand with feet straddling center line "B" (fig. 9.13), facing to the front.
2. Run to the right on the command "Go", touch line "A" with right hand. Turn, facing the front, off the right foot.
3. Run to the left to line "C", touch with left hand, and turn pushing off left foot.
4. Finish by crossing the center line "B".

Speed, Power, Agility, and Endurance Drills 127

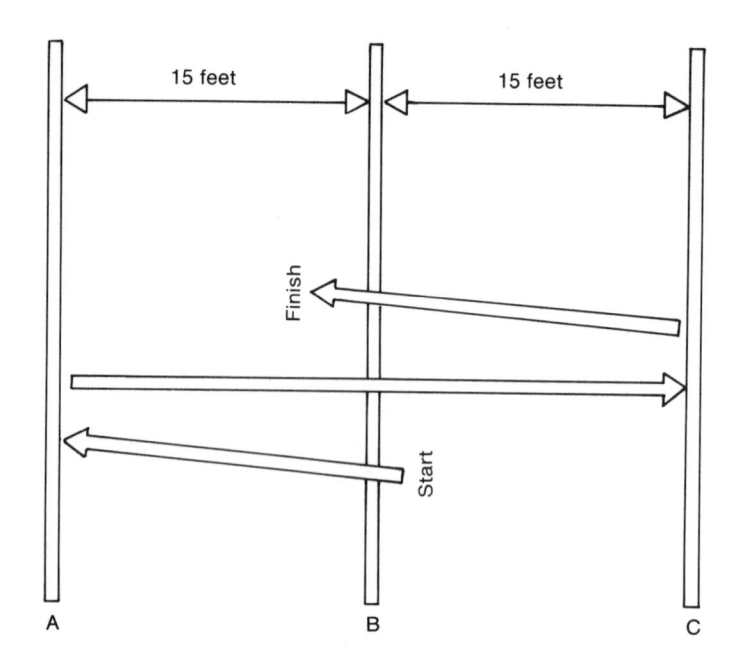

Figure 9.13
Pro Agility Run

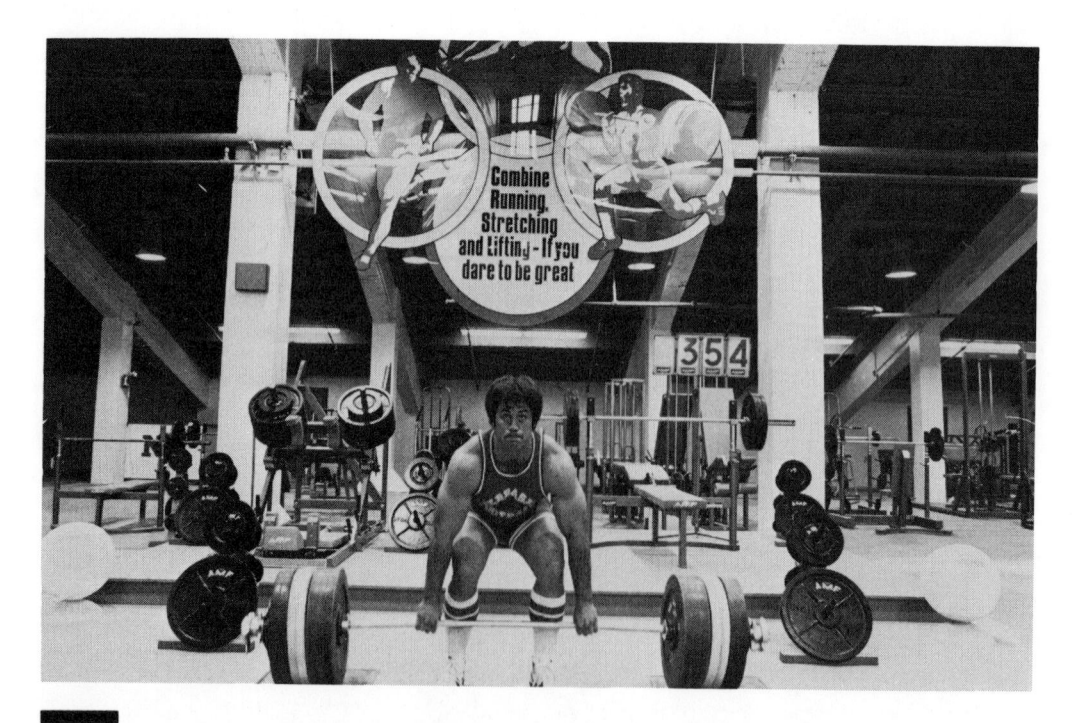

Figure 9.14
"Combine Running, Stretching and Lifting—If You Dare to Be Great"

128 Chapter Nine

Endurance

Endurance is the ability of your muscles to continue to contract without fatiguing. Athletes often fail to realize the importance of training for endurance in their sport. Fatigue has a lot to do with the efficiency of the heart and lungs. In chapter 3 we saw how endurance training can be divided into anaerobic and aerobic conditioning.

Two different methods are used to train for anaerobic and aerobic endurance. Anaerobic conditioning is done by running short, intense sprints, with a rest period in between the workouts. Before starting an anaerobic program, you should first build a base by doing aerobic training. Aerobic conditioning is done by doing long, slow, distance training. If you are trying to gain weight, you should run after you lift so the running doesn't interfere with your strength program. If you are trying to lose weight, you should run before you lift. Many lifters overlook running; many runners do not lift. In the University of Nebraska Strength Complex there is a huge sign that puts it very clearly. It says, "Combine Running, Stretching and Lifting—If You Dare to Be Great."

Aerobic Conditioning for Endurance

Long, slow distance running (or similar activity such as swimming, etc.) is the most popular method of increasing endurance. This method uses the gradual progression of work. Start easy if you are just a beginning runner; walk if necessary. Continue to the next level only when you can run the required times comfortably. Otherwise stay on Level I as long as necessary. Once Level VI has been reached, attempt to increase the distance you can run in twenty minutes each workout. The workouts should be strenuous enough to get a training effect, but not so difficult as to cause exhaustion. Remember, this is only part of your daily workout.

Aerobic Conditioning Program (Tuesday and Friday)

Level	Tuesday	Friday
I	10-minute run	10-minute run
II	12-minute run	12-minute run
III	14-minute run	14-minute run
IV	16-minute run	16-minute run
V	18-minute run	18-minute run
VI	20-minute run	20-minute run

Anaerobic Conditioning for Endurance

NOTE: Before starting on an anaerobic program, first go through the six-level aerobic conditioning program to build your base.

The sprint training, or anaerobic program, also builds for six levels. Once you feel comfortable at Level I, advance to other levels until your competitive season begins.

This program consists of two methods of training—acceleration sprints and interval sprints.

Acceleration Sprints

These can be best accomplished on a football field, or an area one hundred yards long, with markers every twenty yards. One repetition consists of one length of the field. Begin at the goal line; build up speed gradually for twenty yards; sprint twenty yards; ease up for twenty yards; sprint twenty yards. The last twenty yards should be an easy jog into the end zone. You then rest thirty seconds, and repeat the procedure for the required number of repetitions.

Interval Sprints

These are sprints in which repetition is done at maximum speed for a certain distance, followed by a specified recovery period. A wristwatch that accounts for the seconds will probably work best for timing the recovery. After each set, a rest period is allowed.

Anaerobic Program (Tuesday and Friday)

Level	Activity	Repetitions	Rest Intervals
I	Acceleration sprints	10	30 seconds
II	Accleration sprints	8	30 seconds
	Rest 3 minutes		
	Interval sprints—Set 1	10×20 yards	15 seconds
III	Acceleration sprints	6	30 seconds
	Rest 3 minutes		
	Interval sprints—Set 1	5×20 yards	15 seconds
	Rest 2 minutes		
	Interval sprints—Set 2	5×40 yards	20 seconds
IV	Acceleration sprints	4	30 seconds
	Rest 2½ minutes		
	Interval sprints—Set 1	5×20 yards	15 seconds
	Rest 2 minutes		
	Interval sprints—Set 2	5×40 yards	20 seconds
	Rest 2 minutes		
	Interval sprints—Set 3	2×60 yards	30 seconds
V	Acceleration sprints	2	30 seconds
	Rest 2 minutes		
	Interval sprints—Set 1	10×10 yards	10 seconds
	Rest 1 minute		
	Interval sprints—Set 2	5×20 yards	15 seconds
	Rest 2 minutes		
	Interval sprints—Set 3	5×40 yards	20 seconds
	Rest 2 minutes		
	Interval sprints—Set 4	2×60 yards	30 seconds

Level	Activity	Repetitions	Rest Intervals
VI	Acceleration sprints	2	30 seconds
	Rest 2 minutes		
	Interval sprints—Set 1	10×10 yards	10 seconds
	Rest 1 minute		
	Interval sprints—Set 2	10×20 yards	15 seconds
	Rest 2 minutes		
	Interval sprints—Set 3	5×40 yards	20 seconds
	Rest 2 minutes		
	Interval sprints—Set 4	2×60 yards	30 seconds

Many times when an athlete's progress begins to slow down, he or she attempts to train harder in hopes of regaining lost strength or conditioning, ending up shocking the body, losing strength or size, and getting depressed. If you feel you have reached a training plateau, the best solution is to back off on your training so that your body can recuperate. Concentrate on the major exercises and drills only; be sure to get adequate rest; eat good nutritional meals.

Recommended Six-Week Conditioning Program

This is a recommended six-week program that will help you develop into the best athlete that you can possibly be. It integrates the components of strength, speed, power, agility, and endurance necessary to become a great athlete.

Be sure to follow these guidelines:

1. Proper form is critical. Perform each exercise and drill as described in this book.

2. Begin with Week #1, and don't progress faster than the schedule allows. If one week is difficult, stay at that week until you are able to do it easily.

3. Do the daily program in the order it is listed.

4. Do not work out when injured. Consult a trainer or therapist to determine which exercises and drills you might be able to do that won't affect your injury.

Table 9.9
Six-Week Conditioning Schedule—Week One

Program Component	Activity	Repetitions
Monday		
Stretch	8-minute routine	—
Agility	Drill #1 Shuttle run	4
Speed	Drill #1 High knees	4 × 10 yards
	Drill #2 Heel ups	2 × 10 yards
Lifting	Bench press	10
	Incline press	10
	Squat, hip sled, or lunge	10
	Leg extension	10
	Leg curl	10
	Sit-up	10
Tuesday		
Stretch	8-minute routine	
Endurance—Level I		
Aerobic *or* Anaerobic	10-minute run	
	Acceleration sprints	10 (30-second rest intervals)
Lifting	Upright row	10
	Military press	10
	Lateral raise	10
	Bent-over raise	10
	Curl	10
	Tricep extension	10

Table 9.9—*Continued*

Program Component	Activity	Repetitions
Thursday		
Stretch	8-minute routine	
Agility	Drill #2 NE agility	4
Speed	Drill #1 High knees	4 × 10 yards
	Drill #3 Ankle flips	2 × 10 yards
Power	Drill #1 Bounding	2 × 40 yards
Lifting	Bench press	10
	Incline press	10
	Squat, hip sled, or lunge	10
	Leg extension	10
	Leg curl	10
	Sit-up	10
Friday		
Stretch	8-minute routine	
Endurance—Level I		
Aerobic *or* Anaerobic	10-minute run	
	Acceleration sprints	10 (30-second rest intervals)
Lifting	Upright row	10
	Military press	10
	Lateral raise	10
	Bent-over raise	10
	Curl	10
	Tricep extension	10

Table 9.10
Six-Week Conditioning Schedule—Week Two

Program Component	Activity	Repetitions
Monday		
Stretch	8-minute routine	
Agility	Drill #3 Pro agility	4
Speed	Drill #1 High knees	4 × 10 yards
	Drill #2 Heel ups	2 × 10 yards
	Drill #3 Ankle flips	2 × 10 yards
Power	Drill #1 Bounding	2 × 40 yards
	Drill #2 Long jump	5 jumps
Lifting	Bench press	12
	Incline press	12
	Squat, hip sled, or lunge	12
	Leg extension	12
	Leg curl	12
	Sit-up	12
Tuesday		
Stretch	8-minute routine	
Endurance—Level II		
Aerobic *or* Anaerobic	12-minute run	
	Accelerations sprints	8 (30 second rest intervals)
	3-minute rest	
	Interval sprints—Set 1	10 × 20 yards (15 second rest intervals)
Lifting	Upright row	12
	Military press	12
	Lateral raise	12
	Bent-over raise	12
	Curl	12
	Tricep extension	12

Table 9.10—*Continued*

Program Component	Activity	Repetitions
Thursday		
Stretch	8-minute routine	
Agility	Drill #1 Shuttle run	2
	Drill #2 NE agility	2
Speed drills	Drill #1 High knees	4 × 10 yards
	Drill #2 Heel ups	2 × 10 yards
	Drill #3 Ankle flips	2 × 10 yards
Power	Drill #1 Bounding	2 × 40 yards
	Drill # 2 Long jump	5 jumps
Lifting	Bench press	12
	Incline press	12
	Squat, hip sled, or lunge	12
	Leg extension	12
	Leg curl	12
	Sit-up	12
Friday		
Stretch	8-minute routine	
Endurance—Level II	12-minute run	
Aerobic *or* Anaerobic	Acceleration sprints	8 (30 second rest intervals)
	3-minute rest	
	Interval sprints—Set 1	10 × 20 yards (15 second rest intervals)
Lifting	Upright row	12
	Military press	12
	Lateral raise	12
	Bent-over raise	12
	Curl	12
	Tricep extension	12

Table 9.11
Six-Week Conditioning Schedule—Week Three

Program Component	Activity	Repetitions
Monday		
Stretch	8-minute routine	
Agility	Drill #1 Shuttle run	2
	Drill #3 Pro agility	2
Speed	Drill #1 High knees	2 × 10 yards
	Drill #2 Heel ups	2 × 10 yards
	Drill #3 Ankle flips	2 × 10 yards
	Drill #4–5 Form starts	5 × 10 yards
Power	Drill #1 Bounding	2 × 40 yards
	Drill #2 Long jump	3 jumps
	Drill #3A Power jumps	2 × 5 jumps
Lifting	Bench press	15
	Incline press	15
	Squat, hip sled, or lunge	15
	Leg extension	15
	Leg curl	15
	Sit-up	15
Tuesday		
Stretch	8-minute routine	
Endurance—Level III Aerobic *or* Anaerobic	14-minute run	
	Acceleration sprints	6 (30-second rest intervals)
	3-minute rest	
	Interval sprints—Set 1	5 × 20 yards (15-second rest intervals)
	2-minute rest	
	Interval sprints—Set 2	5 × 40 yards (15-second rest intervals)
Lifting	Upright row	15
	Military press	15
	Lateral raise	15
	Bent-over raise	15
	Curl	15
	Tricep extension	15

136   Chapter Nine

Table 9.11—*Continued*

Program Component	Activity	Repetitions
Thursday		
Stretch	8-minute routine	
Agility	Drill #2 NE agility	2
	Drill #3 Pro agility	2
Speed	Drill #1 High knees	2 × 10 yards
	Drill #2 Heel ups	2 × 10 yards
	Drill #3 Ankle flips	2 × 10 yards
	Drill #4–5 Form starts	5 × 10 yards
Power	Drill #1 Bounding	2 × 40 yards
	Drill #2 Long jump	3 jumps
	Drill #3B Speed jumps	4 × 20 yards
Lifting	Bench press	15
	Incline press	15
	Squat, hip sled, or lunge	15
	Leg extension	15
	Leg curl	15
	Sit-up	15
Friday		
Stretch	8-minute routine	
Endurance—Level III Aerobic *or* Anaerobic	14-minute run	
	Acceleration sprints	6 (30-second rest intervals)
	3-minute rest	
	Interval sprints—Set 1	5 × 20 yards (15 second rest intervals)
	2-minute rest	
	Interval Sprints—Set 2	5 × 40 yards (15-second rest intervals)
Lifting	Upright row	15
	Military press	15
	Lateral raise	15
	Bent-over raise	15
	Curl	15
	Tricep extension	15

**Table 9.12
Six-Week Conditioning Schedule—Week Four**

Program Component	Activity	Repetitions
Monday		
Stretch	8-minute routine	
Agility	Drill #1 Shuttle run	3
	Drill #2 NE Agility	3
Speed	Drill #1 High knees	2 × 10 yards
	Drill #2 Heel ups	2 × 10 yards
	Drill #3 Ankle flips	2 × 10 yards
	Drill #4–5 Form starts	5 × 10 yards
	Drill #6 Form sprints	3 × 50 yards
Power	Drill #1 Bounding	2 × 40 yards
	Drill #3A Power jumps	2 × 5 jumps
	Drill #4 Single leg hops	5 hops (each leg)
Lifting	Bench press	2 sets (15/10)
	Incline press	2 sets (15/10)
	Squat, hip sled, or lunge	2 sets (15/10)
	Leg extension	2 sets (15/10)
	Leg curl	2 sets (15/10)
	Sit-up	2 sets (15/10)
Tuesday		
Stretch	8-minute routine	
Endurance—Level IV Aerobic *or* Anaerobic	16-minute run	
	Acceleration sprints—Set 1	4 (30-second rest intervals)
	2½-minute rest	
	Interval sprints—Set 1	5 × 20 yards (15-second rest intervals)
	2-minute rest	
	Interval sprints—Set 2	5 × 40 yards (20-second rest intervals)
	2-minute rest	
	Interval sprints—Set 3	2 × 60 yards (30-second rest intervals)
Lifting	Upright row	2 sets (15/10)
	Military press	2 sets (15/10)
	Lateral raise	2 sets (15/10)
	Bent-over raise	2 sets (15/10)
	Curl	2 sets (15/10)
	Tricep extension	2 sets (15/10)

Table 9.12—*Continued*

Program Component	Activity	Repetitions
Thursday		
Stretch	8-minute routine	
Agility	Drill #1 Shuttle run	3
	Drill #3 Pro agility	2
Speed	Drill #1 High knees	2 × 10 yards
	Drill #2 Heel ups	2 × 10 yards
	Drill #3 Ankle flips	2 × 10 yards
	Drill #4–5 Form starts	5 × 10 yards
	Drill #6 Form sprints	5 × 50 yards
Power	Drill #1 Bounding	2 × 40 yards
	Drill #3B Speed jumps	2 × 20 yards
	Drill #4 Single leg hops	5 hops (each leg)
Lifting	Bench press	2 sets (15/10)
	Incline press	2 sets (15/10)
	Squat, hip sled, or lunge	2 sets (15/10)
	Leg extension	2 sets (15/10)
	Leg curl	2 sets (15/10)
	Sit-up	2 sets (15/10)
Friday		
Stretch	8-minute routine	
Endurance—Level IV Aerobic *or* Anaerobic	16-minute run	
	Acceleration sprints	4 (30-second rest intervals)
	2½-minute rest	
	Interval sprints—Set 1	5 × 20 yards (15-second rest intervals)
	2-minute rest	
	Interval sprints—Set 2	5 × 40 yards (20-second rest intervals)
	2-minute rest	
	Interval sprints—Set 3	2 × 60 yards (30-second rest intervals)
Lifting	Upright row	2 sets (15/10)
	Military press	2 sets (15/10)
	Lateral raise	2 sets (15/10)
	Bent-over raise	2 sets (15/10)
	Curl	2 sets (15/10)
	Tricep extension	2 sets (15/10)

Table 9.13
Six-Week Conditioning Schedule—Week Five

Program Component	Activity	Repetitions
Monday		
Stretch	8-minute routine	
Agility	Drill #2 NE agility	3
	Drill #3 Pro agility	3
Speed	Drill #1 High knees	2 × 10 yards
	Drill #2 Heel ups	2 × 10 yards
	Drill #3 Ankle flips	2 × 10 yards
	Drill #4–5 Form starts	5 × 10 yards
	Drill #6 Form sprints	3 × 50 yards
Power	Drill #1 Bounding	2 × 40 yards
	Drill #3A Power jumps	2 × 5 jumps
	Drill #4 Single leg hops	5 hops (each leg)
	Drill #5A 10/10 hopping	2 × 40 yards
Lifting	Bench press	2 sets (15/12)
	Incline press	2 sets (15/12)
	Squat, hip sled, or lunge	2 sets (15/12)
	Leg extension	2 sets (15/12)
	Leg curl	2 sets (15/12)
	Sit-up	2 sets (15/12)
Tuesday		
Stretch	8-minute routine	
Endurance—Level V		
Aerobic *or* Anaerobic	18-minute run	
	Accleration sprints	2 (30-second rest intervals)
	2-minute rest	
	Interval sprints—Set 1	10 × 10 yards (10-second rest intervals)
	1-minute rest	
	Interval sprints—Set 2	5 × 20 yards (15-second rest intervals)
	2-minute rest	
	Interval sprints—Set 3	5 × 40 yards (20-second rest intervals)
	2-minute rest	
	Interval sprints—Set 4	2 × 60 yards (30-second rest intervals)
Lifting	Upright row	2 sets (15/12)
	Military press	2 sets (15/12)
	Lateral raise	2 sets (15/12)
	Bent-over raise	2 sets (15/12)
	Curl	2 sets (15/12)
	Tricep extension	2 sets (15/12)

Table 9.13—*Continued*

Program Component	Activity	Repetitions
Thursday		
Stretch	8-minute routine	
Agility	Drill #2 NE agility	3
	Drill #3 Pro agility	3
Speed	Drill #1 High knees	2 × 10 yards
	Drill #2 Heel ups	2 × 10 yards
	Drill #3 Ankle flips	2 × 10 yards
	Drill #4–5 Form starts	5 × 10 yards
	Drill #6 Form sprints	5 × 50 yards
Power	Drill #1 Bounding	2 × 40 yards
	Drill #3B Power jumps	2 × 20 yards
	Drill #4 Single leg hops	5 hops (each leg)
	Drill #5B Power hops	2 × 5 hops (each leg)
Lifting	Bench press	2 sets (15/12)
	Incline press	2 sets (15/12)
	Squat, hip sled, or lunge	2 sets (15/12)
	Leg extension	2 sets (15/12)
	Leg curl	2 sets (15/12)
	Sit-up	2 sets (15/12)
Friday		
Stretch	8-minute routine	
Endurance—Level V Aerobic *or* Anaerobic	18-minute run	
	Acceleration sprints	2 (30-second rest intervals)
	2-minute rest	
	Interval sprints—Set 1	10 × 10 yards (10-second rest intervals)
	1-minute rest	
	Interval sprints—Set 2	5 × 20 yards (15-second rest intervals)
	2-minute rest	
	Interval sprints—Set 3	5 × 40 yards (20-second rest intervals)
	2-minute rest	
	Interval sprints—Set 4	2 × 60 yards (30-second rest intervals)
Lifting	Upright row	2 sets (15/12)
	Military press	2 sets (15/12)
	Lateral raise	2 sets (15/12)
	Bent-over raise	2 sets (15/12)
	Curl	2 sets (15/12)
	Tricep extension	2 sets (15/12)

Table 9.14
Six-Week Conditioning Schedule—Week Six

Program Component	Activity	Repetitions
Monday		
Stretch	8-minute routine	
Agility	Drill #1 Shuttle run	2
	Drill #2 NE agility	2
	Drill #3 Pro agility	2
Speed	Drill #1 High knees	2 × 10 yards
	Drill #2 Heel ups	2 × 10 yards
	Drill #3 Ankle flips	2 × 10 yards
	Drill #4–5 Form starts	5 × 10 yards
	Drill #6 Form sprints	5 × 50 yards
Power	Drill #1 Bounding	2 × 40 yards
	Drill #3A Power jumps	2 × 5 jumps
	Drill #3B Speed jumps	2 × 20 yards
	Drill #5A 10/10 hopping	2 × 40 yards
	Drill #5B Power hops	2 × 5 hops (each leg)
Lifting	Bench press	2 sets (15/15)
	Incline press	2 sets (15/15)
	Squat, hip sled, or lunge	2 sets (15/15)
	Leg extension	2 sets (15/15)
	Leg curl	2 sets (15/15)
	Sit-up	2 sets (15/15)
Tuesday		
Stretch	8-minute routine	
Endurance—Level VI Aerobic *or* Anaerobic	20-minute run	
	Acceleration sprints	2 (30-second rest intervals)
	2-minute rest	
	Interval sprints—Set 1	10 × 10 yards (10-second rest intervals)
	1-minute rest	
	Interval sprints—Set 2	10 × 20 yards (15-second rest intervals)
	2-minute rest	
	Interval sprints—Set 3	5 × 40 yards (20-second rest intervals)
	2-minute rest	
	Interval sprints—Set 4	2 × 60 yards (30-second rest intervals)
Lifting	Upright row	2 sets (15/15)
	Military press	2 sets (15/15)
	Lateral raise	2 sets (15/15)
	Bent-over raise	2 sets (15/15)
	Curl	2 sets (15/15)
	Tricep extension	2 sets (15/15)

Table 9.14—*Continued*

Program Component	Activity	Repetitions
Thursday		
Stretch	8-minute routine	
Agility	Drill #1 Shuttle run	2
	Drill #2 NE agility	2
	Drill #3 Pro agility	2
Speed	Drill #1 High knees	2 × 10 yards
	Drill #2 Heel ups	2 × 10 yards
	Drill #3 Ankle flips	2 × 10 yards
	Drill #4–5 Form starts	5 × 10 yards
	Drill #6 Form sprints	5 × 50 yards
Power	Drill #1 Bounding	2 × 40 yards
	Drill #3A Power jumps	2 × 5 jumps
	Drill #3B Speed jumps	2 × 20 yards
	Drill #5A 10/10 hopping	2 × 40 yards
	Drill #5B Power hops	2 × 5 hops (each leg)
Lifting	Bench press	2 sets (15/15)
	Incline press	2 sets (15/15)
	Squat, hip sled, or lunge	2 sets (15/15)
	Leg extension	2 sets (15/15)
	Leg curl	2 sets (15/15)
	Sit-up	2 sets (15/15)
Friday		
Stretch	8-minute routine	
Endurance—Level VI Aerobic *or* Anaerobic	20-minute run	
	Acceleration sprints	2 (30-second rest intervals)
	2-minute rest	
	Interval sprints—Set 1	10 × 10 yards (10-second rest intervals)
	1-minute rest	
	Interval sprints—Set 2	10 × 20 yards (15-second rest intervals)
	2-minute rest	
	Interval sprints—Set 3	5 × 40 yards (20-second rest intervals)
	2-minute rest	
	Interval sprints—Set 4	2 × 60 yards (30-second rest intervals)
Lifting	Upright row	2 sets (15/15)
	Military press	2 sets (15/15)
	Lateral raise	2 sets (15/15)
	Bent-over raise	2 sets (15/15)
	Curl	2 sets (15/15)
	Tricep extension	2 sets (15/15)

CHAPTER TEN

How to Keep Your Body Strong

Unfortunately your body never stays the same. It is either changing for the better (improvement), or it is getting worse. Today's society provides plenty of roadblocks along your path to success. You have the ability to avoid these roadblocks. Some of the most notorious of these are overeating, smoking, drinking alcohol, and drugs. They can not only hold back your progress, but could end your athletic career. Take charge of your life and don't let any of these obstacles prevent you from reaching your athletic goals.

Don't Overeat

A sensible diet is an important contribution to your overall performance. A balanced diet that includes foods from all of the four major groups—meat, dairy, fruits and vegetables, breads and cereals—will provide you with the energy you need for exercise and recovery.

Overeating each day means you will gain weight in the form of fat that collects beneath your skin. People who are fat when they are young tend to remain fat all their adult lives. Some of the consequences are heart disease, kidney disease, and high blood pressure. Sagging fat is not appealing, and it will not help your performance as an athlete.

Figure 10.1
Balance

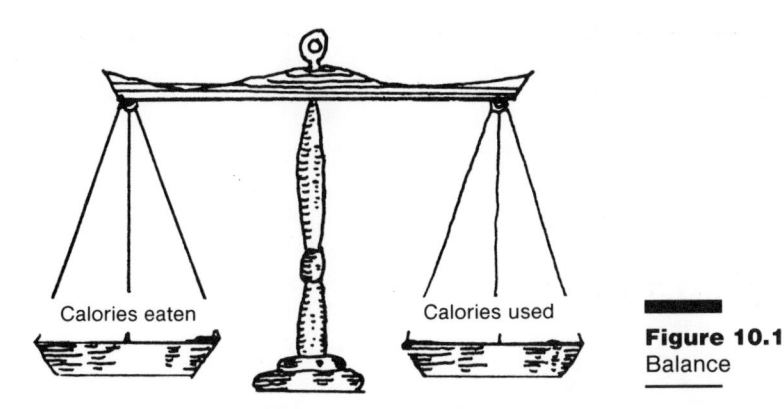

Food is made up of calories. Some types of food have more calories than other types. For example, six ounces of hamburger has 490 calories, while six ounces of green beans has twenty-five calories. Your body uses these calories in the form of energy to perform various functions such as work, exercise, and keeping the body warm. If your daily intake of calories balances with the number of calories your body uses each day, then your body weight will pretty much remain the same. If you eat more calories than you use up in a day, a gain in body weight will take place. If your body uses more calories than you have eaten, a loss in body weight will result.

Your body has to use three-thousand-five-hundred calories to lose one pound. In view of the amount of activity it would take for you to burn off each pound of fat, something more than merely exercising is called for. Smart dieting is the key to losing fat, while exercise is an aid. If you are fat you should strive to eliminate your excess body fat over a long period of time, rather than by a potentially dangerous crash diet.

Most young athletes are actually trying to gain weight, rather than lose weight. They have trouble eating enough calories each day through their normal three meals to offset the calories they burn up by working out.

If you want to gain weight, and are involved in an exercise program, then you must increase your normal caloric intake as required by your age, height, and body build. This is why athletes in training who are trying to gain weight are advised by team physicians or trainers to supplement their training table diet by drinking additional calories, usually in the form of liquid nutriments.

If you are trying to gain body weight, you may want to try the new Pro-Gain powdered weight gain formula (fig. 10.2) to provide your body with the nutrients that your stronger, more calorie-demanding muscles require each day. This is taken to afford the body additional calories to effect a gain in weight. (Send for more information from the address in the back of the book). Of course, this weight gain supplement is to be taken in conjunction with a strength training program.

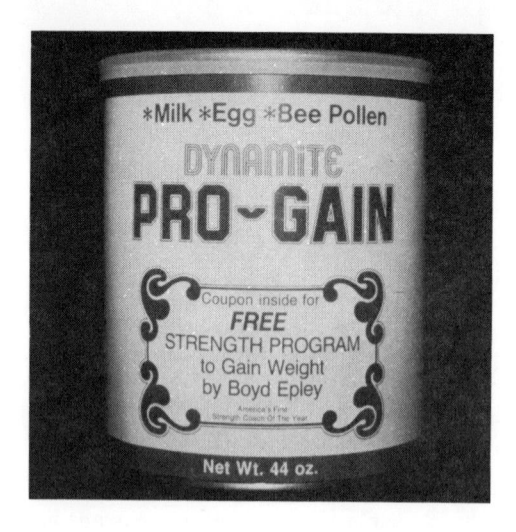

Figure 10.2
Pro-Gain

I should point out that the programs for gaining weight pertain mainly to men. Most women can dramatically increase their strength levels through a lifting program, but gain very little muscle size or body weight due to a difference in hormones.

Don't Smoke

It is impossible for any athlete who smokes to be in top physical condition, because correct breathing during exercise is hampered by smoking. Breathing is accomplished by the expansion and contraction of a large muscle called the diaphragm, as well as the expansion and contraction of the chest muscles with the aid of the diaphragm. The entire efficiency of the breathing apparatus depends upon the strength and tone of the diaphragm and chest muscles. Like all other muscles, these become strong and active through increased exercise.

Exercise forces the lungs to handle more air per minute, purify more blood per minute, and remove more waste from the blood per minute. Smoke clogs your lungs, and this carbon monoxide works to prevent oxygen from entering your blood stream. When you exercise, your lungs can't supply all of the oxygen needed by your muscles. Fatigue sets in and hampers your performance.

Although it may take a few workouts for beginners to perfect the correct breathing pattern, it is essential that breathing during exercise be performed properly. Inhale as you begin to lift. Advanced athletes hold their breath while performing a repetition. This stabilizes the chest muscles, allowing them to exert greater force on the weight being lifted. Do not hold the breath for more than one repetition. No matter what the starting exercise position, inhalation takes place at that point. The breath is then held until near completion of the repetition, when the air is forcibly exhaled. If you have ever had problems with headaches, you should not hold your breath at all while exercising.

Don't Take Drugs or Drink Alcohol

Alcohol affects your physical performance in the same way that cigarettes do—it makes it difficult for hardworking muscles to receive oxygen. Advanced cases of alcohol consumption can lead to liver disease, loss of brain cells, and even death. Alcohol also has an impact on the heart muscle. A brief drinking spree by an apparently healthy individual can result in premature heart disease, or a total loss of rhythmic beating in the chambers of the heart.

Drinking alcohol is one of the biggest problems the young athlete has to overcome. Most young athletes think they are pretty tough and can handle a few drinks. What they don't realize is that some people simply cannot tolerate any alcohol without becoming an alcoholic. Sure, there are some of your friends who will never become alcoholics, but 10 percent of Americans are alcoholics. It doesn't matter how big or how strong or how tough you are.

Let me tell you about a football player named Bob Newton. He was 6'4" and 275 pounds back in 1970, and was the strongest football player Nebraska had at the time, with a 375-pound bench press and a 305-pound incline press. I was very proud when Bob was named All-American, because he was the first All-American player I had worked with in my newly-formed strength training program. He was drafted by the Chicago Bears, and they got one tough rookie lineman. He was so tough that he earned the respect of the veterans, and was invited to party with them after the first game. He was really excited about this because rookies were not usually included when the veterans got together to drink. Big Bob knew he had drunk a little more than he should have to drive a car, but when one of the veterans asked the rookie to go for more beer around 5:00 in the morning, Bob went. He was arrested

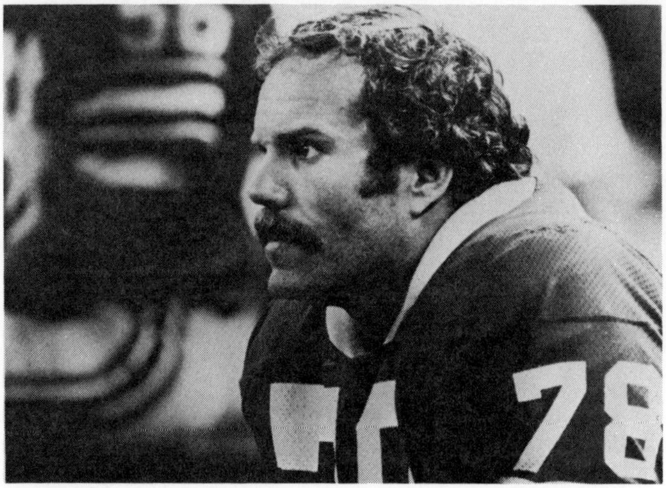

Figure 10.3
Bob Newton

for drunk driving, and his coach from the Chicago Bears had to come to the police station to bail him out. Bob has been arrested for drunk driving five times since then, and was kicked out of professional football after coming to a football meeting drunk. Bob Newton says:

> When I was a player at the University of Nebraska, the way I drank was accepted normal behavior. The guys that I usually associated with on the team drank like I did, and if they didn't, then I didn't hang around with them. At that time I really didn't feel as if I had a drinking problem. I based all my fun and joy around drinking, and since I was performing well on the field, I didn't think the alcohol was interfering with my life. It wasn't until after being traded to the Seattle Seahawks years later than I found out what had started in college as a means to have some fun had turned into a full-fledged addiction at age 33. I was released from the Seahawks because my performance was affected by my consumption of alcohol and drugs.
>
> I think the lowest point of my life came when Dick Coury, the head coach of the Boston Breakers of the USFL, finally ended my professional career when he had to kick me off the team because I was too drunk to practice. He said, "Bob, you are going to end up on skid row unless you take care of this alcohol problem."
>
> Basically, I was failing to find constructive alternatives socially and psychologically to deal with life without alcohol. Only because of God-given ability was my performance on the field still getting by. I failed to recognize that I had a problem that was deeply rooted in me; it wasn't going to go away and I couldn't just wish it away.
>
> The way I was drinking made it very easy for me to get into the groove of using other drugs such as cocaine and marijuana. The first time I took cocaine I found out I could drink more, and it was great; I just kept drinking and did not seem to get drunk. But what I failed to realize was that cocaine was promoting my drunkenness a lot farther, and I would get to the point where I would be staggering, slobbering, slurring my words, with my eyes barely open, and still with a drink in my hand. That shows you how powerless I was over alcohol and drugs.
>
> The money I spent on cocaine, marijuana, and alcohol was outrageous, but I always could point to somebody worse than me. I know of several veterans who played 15–16 years of pro-football, including the Super Bowl, and they have ended up penniless because of alcohol and drugs.
>
> At age 33 I was left without football; all I had was myself to look at, and I didn't see anything. I didn't see any personal growth. I was almost a vegetable. I had nothing inside. Fortunately the grace of God led me to a rehabilitation center for alcohol and drug abuse. I was there 28 days, and I finally learned what I was dealing with.
>
> I always had this macho feeling that I was tough and no bottle of beer was going to control me. So after 14 years of unmanageability in my life, financial instability, a divorce, and being kicked off my team, I finally had to admit that alcohol was tougher than I was. I feel lucky to be alive.

Many professional teams have now incorporated drug testing into their annual team physicals, and more teams will follow. Colleges have also begun drug testing to prevent athletes from ruining their lives by thinking they can handle drugs.

Marijuana

Some young people think marijuana is not harmful, but it is. THC, the major psychoactive substance in marijuana, tends to accumulate in the brain, sex glands, and fatty tissues of the body. There is evidence that marijuana may cause irreversible damage to the brain if used for several years. Young athletes cannot afford this deterioration of mental functioning. The symptoms associated with marijuana use include dullness, lack of motivation, impairment of judgment, poor memory, and slowed speech.[2]

Cocaine

The reaction to cocaine at first is laughter, excitement, restlessness, and habitual talking. If use is continued, the initial mild reaction is followed by a very destructive progression of symptoms that lead to death. These symptoms include emotional instability, increased pulse rate, convulsions, circulatory failure, respiratory failure, paralysis, and death.[3]

Don't Use Steroids

Both males and females produce male and female hormones. The male hormone is known as testosterone, which causes the body to retain nitrogen. Nitrogen is a part of the chemical structure of amino acids. These are the building blocks for your body, and enhance the muscle protein necessary for muscular development. This feature of testosterone is called its *anabolic action,* which refers to the building action in contrast to the *catabolic action,* which is a tearing down function. When male athletes take anabolic steroids, the steroids act like testosterone in the endocrine system. They inhibit the pituitary gland (located at the base of the brain), which controls sexual development. They may affect the pituitary's ability to stimulate the testicles in the way that birth control pills affect the pituitary's ability to suppress ovulation in women. The list of undesirable complications associated with the use of steroids is long: acne, inhibition of testicular function, testicular atrophy, low sperm counts, impotence, breast enlargement, and excessive persistent sexual stimulation. In addition, use of steroids may cause the liver to have difficulty in expelling its bile. Bile may be retained in the small liver cells, which begins a long chain of events leading to liver disease.

Women, too, have used anabolic steroids. The sexual side effects in women include development of masculine characteristics, including an increase in prominent facial hair. This may not go away after use of anabolic steroids is discontinued. Not surprisingly, use of anabolic steroids also affect a woman's menstrual cycle and her voice, and may even induce male pattern baldness.[4]

There is widespread use of anabolic steroids in the strength training field today. These tissue building drugs can have highly undesirable side effects for the young athlete. Adolescents using steroids can end up shorter in stature because the drugs close bone growth plates prematurely. You have only one body. Take the best care of it that you possibly can. Stay away from drugs. You don't need them.

Get Sufficient Sleep

Your body has a greater than average need to be recharged during sleep because it is still growing.

There will always be two processes going on in your body as long as you live. The first, called anabolism, is the building up of cells, tissues, and energy—and the repair and maintenance of body parts. The second, called catabolism, is the tearing down of living tissue, the release of energy, and the creation of waste matter.

Together, anabolism and catabolism are called metabolism. While we are awake, the tearing down process (catabolism) is much faster than the building up process (anabolism). The result is tiredness. The harder we work the more tired we become.

While we are asleep, the process (anabolism) has a chance to recharge your body with new energy and new tissue. You must get at least eight hours of sleep in order for your growing body to get recharged. Even a small loss of sleep will result in general irritability, and could result in illness.

Conclusion

Regardless of how much or how little talent you may possess, you can still become a successful athlete. I have seen average athletes become All-Americans through hard work and a high degree of personal motivation. If you want to accomplish something as an athlete, don't quit until it is accomplished. No matter who you are or how great your athletic talent, you will face adversity. Successful athletes are the ones with the perseverance and the persistence to keep training hard as they struggle toward their goal. No matter how many roadblocks or obstacles are put in their way, they keep going until they reach their goal. If you want to be a champion athlete you must have this burning desire in you to be a winner. This desire must be so great that you are motivated to put in the long hours of training and practice, and make the sacrifices needed to succeed. No reward is greater than your own personal happiness. Happiness will be achieved when you reach your goal. It is amazing how the simple feeling of happiness will motivate you to work harder to achieve even greater goals for yourself. Let each of your lifting sessions and running workouts be stepping stones toward reaching your goal and you will soon experience this tremendous personal satisfaction.

This book can help you by telling you what training needs to be done and how often to do it. But you must supply the rest. Your enthusiasm towards working out is very important. You can't fake enthusiasm day after day, week after week. The workouts will become too long and too hard. You must have the desire, the determination, and the dedication to carry you on to your goal. There are no shortcuts in the world of athletics; only goals to be set and goals to be reached. Naturally, it is more fun to work on your strong points because they are what you do best, but the fastest way to improve your athletic talent is to work on improving your weak areas. You will never reach your full potential if you concentrate only on what you are best at. Turn your weaknesses into your strengths and you will have a new confidence that no one can take away.

You only have one body and you only go through life once. You should feel a sense of guilt if you have not done everything in your power to reach your full potential in life. Athletes have to pay the price, not just when they feel like it, but according to a schedule. Sometimes you have to practice and work out when you would rather be doing something else. It is easy to accept defeat when you know you haven't worked very hard to win, but if you have trained as hard as your schedule dictates, no one knows better than you that you are ready for the competition. Everyone likes to win, but not everyone will prepare to win. Great athletes are the hardest losers because they have trained harder and have more to lose. There are times when you would rather be somewhere else than doing your workouts, but you must force yourself to remain enthusiastic and positive—and force yourself to work harder, even when you might be sad or troubled. This is mental toughness.

The skills gained from hours of training enable you to have mental confidence in yourself. This mental confidence allows you to perform to your fullest. Late in the game, in the last few yards of a race, or when the last points need to be scored, it is the best-conditioned athlete—not necessarily the most talented—who will win. You can't always beat your opponents in talent, but you can beat them in conditioning.

You can get anything out of life you want, if you just keep trying. Sooner or later you will reach your goal. If you get discouraged and quit training, your goal will never be reached, and as you get older and you look back on your life the goals you once had will be just memories. It is one of the saddest things to see people look back on their life and wonder what might have been if they would have worked a little harder. At your age you still have time to set goals and reach for them. It is not where you are now that counts, but where you end up. These training practices and principles will get you headed in the right direction, the rest is up to you. Your work habits will determine your future as an athlete.

Notes

1. Legwold, Gary. 1982. Does lifting weights harm a prepubescent athlete? *The Physician and Sportsmedicine.* 10: 7.

2. Dabney, Anna. 1979. Drugs of abuse—marijuana. *Syva Signal Newsletter.* 3; Nahas, Gabriel G. 1979. *Keep off the grass.* Pergamon Press.

3. Ellis, George M. 1983. Drugs of abuse—cocaine. *Syva Signal Newsletter.* 2.

4. Lamb, L. E. 1984. *The Health Letter.* 23: 9.

Appendix

AMF—American Athletic
200 American Avenue
Jefferson, Iowa 50129

Body Enterprises
P. O. Box 80577
Lincoln, Nebraska 68501

National Strength & Conditioning Association
251 Capitol Beach Blvd.
Lincoln, Nebraska 68508

Glossary

AAU Amateur Athletic Union.
acceleration sprints A type of sprint training characterized by a building up to full speed, then gradually slowing down, and repeating again.
aerobic exercise Exercise in which oxygen is used.
agility The ability to change directions rapidly, maintaining balance without the loss of speed.
agonist A contracting muscle or group of muscles.
AMF American Manufacturing Foundry, a company that manufactures strength and conditioning equipment.
anabolic action Protein building.
anaerobic exercise Exercise without the use of oxygen.

antagonist The muscles on the opposite side of the joint from the muscles being worked. For example, if you are working your biceps, your triceps are the antagonist; if you are working your triceps, your biceps are antagonists.
asthma An allergic disorder that affects respiration.
ATP (adenosine triphosphate) The energy fuel used by the body to contract the muscles.

balanced diet A diet that has the proper balance of fats, carbohydrates, and protein—achieved by eating foods from each of the four basic food groups daily.
balanced program A conditioning program that develops the overall body, working each muscle group equally.

barbell A bar with adjustable, but balanced, weighted disks on each end. Used for strength training exercises.

basic movement skills Skills that can be performed at an early age, such as jumping, catching, and climbing to improve coordination.

body builder A person who develops the physique through a combination of exercise and diet for the purposes of competition and exhibition.

body composition The ratio of lean body mass to body fat.

Body Enterprises A strength and conditioning consulting corporation.

calories A measurement of the energy-producing property of foods.

capillary A small vessel, located between arteries and veins, where exchanges between tissue and blood occur.

cardiovascular endurance The ability of the lungs and heart to take in and transport adequate amounts of oxygen to the working muscles, allowing one to perform activities that involve large muscle masses over long periods of time.

catabolic action Breakdown of complex materials within the body.

collar On barbells, a clamp that secures the plate on the bar.

competition bench A bench press bench with the uprights approximately forty-five inches apart.

conditioning profile A chart used to compare an individual's test results with a control group of the same age, sex, or position to point out strengths and weaknesses.

contraction The shortening of the length of a muscle.

cycling Periodical changes in the number of sets, repetitions, and degree of intensity, to enhance strength gains over a period of time.

desire To long or hope for. To express a wish for.

diaphragm A muscle that aids in the breathing process.

dumbbell A short bar with identical spheres or adjustable weighted disks attached to each end.

epiphyseal plate A layer of cartilage between the end of a long bone and its shaft that allows the bone to increase in length in early adulthood.

epiphysis The end of a long bone, usually larger in diameter than the shaft (the diaphysis). The plural form is *epiphyses*.

fast twitch A muscle fiber characterized by fast contraction time, high anaerobic capacity, and low aerobic capacity. These fibers are best suited for high power activities.

flexibility The ability to move the body parts through their full range of motion.

flexing Contracting a muscle to bring out its size and definition for competition or exhibition.

force The capacity for exerting strength.

full range-of-motion The greatest range possible for a muscle or group of muscles.

hormones Chemical substances secreted into the body fluids by an endocrine gland, which have specific effects on the activities of other cells, tissues, and organs.

hyperextension Extension of a limb to a greater degree than the normal maximal extension.

inhalation Breathing in.

interval sprints A type of sprint training characterized by sprinting at full speed, followed by a specified recovery time, then repeating.

in-season program A program to be used while competing to maintain the strength and conditioning levels that have been achieved by the pre-season program.

joint Point where two bones come together, and act as a hinge.

lactic acid The waste product generated by the body's use of ATP.
lean body mass Your bodyweight minus your body fat.
lifting belt A belt that supports the lower back while lifting.
ligament The band (or sheet) of fibrous tissue that connects bones or cartilage, and serves to strengthen the joint.

major exercise An exercise that directly improves your athletic performance.
metabolism The sum total of the chemical changes that occur in the body.
motivation Anything that impels a person to keep moving toward a goal.
motor unit A group of muscle fibers commonly innervated by one motor nerve.
motor unit recruitment Occurs when the body calls on motor units to do a task. More motor units are recruited to lift heavier poundages.
muscle-bound The enlargement of the muscles to the point that muscle elasticity is reduced, resulting in a negative effect on performance.
muscle fiber An elongated thread-like strand of muscle.
muscle tone Ability of a few motor units to be activated, as necessary, to keep the body from collapsing while in a relaxed state.
muscular endurance The ability to withstand isolated, as well as overall, effects of fatigue on the body during prolonged work.

narrow stance A bench press bench with the uprights approximately sixteen inches apart.
nitrogen A gas that is part of the chemical structure of amino acids.
NSCA National Strength and Conditioning Association. A nonprofit organization that publishes a bimonthly journal to exchange training ideas.

off-season program A program to be used while not competing, to enhance strength and conditioning levels.
Olympic plates Weights that have a 2" diameter center hole, for use with an Olympic bar.

Olympic set A weight set that includes a 7' 2" inch revolving bar, and plates that have a 2" diameter hole.
one-hundred-ten-pound set A standard bar with locks, in addition to an assortment of 10-, 5-, 2½-, and 1¼-pound standard plates that total 110 pounds.
overload To work harder than the body is accustomed to.
overtraining A state of reduced muscle size and strength, which occurs as a result of working at too high an intensity, or not allowing enough recovery time over a long period of time.

plyometrics A type of training that develops explosive power.
poundage The amount of weight used.
power Application of maximum force in the shortest period of time possible.
power lifting A competitive situation in which individuals try to lift as much as possible for one repetition each on three exercises: squat, bench press, and deadlift.
pro gain A powdered weight gain drink that is balanced in fats, carbohydrates, and proteins.
progress chart A chart for recording your workout poundages and repetitions.
puberty The time of life when the secondary sex characteristics begin to appear, usually occuring between the ages of ten and fifteen years.

recovery The time necessary for the muscles to rebuild themselves, after being torn down during a workout.
repetitions (reps) The number of times you repeat an exercise or movement.
rest between sets The amount of time taken between the conclusion of one set and the beginning of the next set.
rest intervals Duration of rest between work bouts.

slow twitch A muscle fiber characterized by slow contracting time, high aerobic capacity, and low anaerobic capacity. These fibers are best suited for endurance activities.

speed The distance covered per unit of time.
split routine A program that works half of the body parts on certain days of the week, and the other half on the remaining days.
spotter Person who aids the lifter, if help is needed.
squat cage Squat uprights, with a lower safety rack that prevents the athlete from getting hurt if unable to stand up with the weight.
standard bar A solid 1" bar, either 5 or 6 feet in length.
standard plates Weights that have a 1⅛" diameter hole for use with a standard bar.
strength The degree of ability to apply or resist force.
strength training A type of training that involves an increase in strength to enhance athletic performance.
stretching routine A prescribed set of exercises to increase flexibility.
stride frequency Number of strides taken per second.
stride length The distance covered in one stride.
supplementary exercise An exercise that indirectly improves athletic performance.

techniques The proper method of performance for an exercise or drill.
tendons A fibrous band, or cord, that attaches a muscle to bone.
training goals The desired performance levels an athlete is working toward.
training load The poundage used for workouts.
training plateau State attained when strength gains peak and level off.
Tuflex A special, non-slick, high-density, rubber flooring that provides good footing and withstands hard pounding.

UPI (United Press International) Annually sponsors a poll of the coaches of a particular sport to recognize outstanding athletes.
USFL (United States Football League) A professional football league.

warm-up sets The performance of the exact movement of an exercise, but using lighter weight, for six to eight repetitions before exercising with heavy weights.
weight lifting A competitive sport in which an individual trys to lift as much weight as possible.
weight training A type of training that results in increased strength for improvement in fitness.

Index

A
AAU, 13, 157
acceleration sprints, 130, 131, 157
aerobic exercise, 24, 129, 132–134, 157
agility, 8, 11, 15, 105, 107, 117, 126–128, 157
agonist, 53, 157
AMF, 15, 16, 29, 35–38, 76, 80, 106, 155, 157
anabolic action, 149, 150, 157
anaerobic exercise, 24, 129, 130, 132–143, 157
antagonist, 53, 157
asthma, 8, 10, 157
ATP (adenosine triphosphate), 21, 24, 26, 157

B
balanced diet, 5, 41, 144, 157
balanced program, 19, 41, 77–79, 97, 98, 157
barbell, 8, 30, 62–104, 158
basic movement skills, 2, 158

body builder, 9, 10, 12, 13, 158
body composition, 26, 145, 158
Body Enterprises, 15, 29, 31, 38, 155, 158

C
calories, 145, 158
capillary, 21, 158
cardiovascular endurance, 15, 158
catabolic action, 149, 150, 158
collar, 4, 158
competition bench, 62, 158
conditioning profile, 109–116, 158
contraction, 1, 21, 25, 51, 53, 59, 98, 146, 158
cycling, 6, 40, 41, 42, 43, 48, 50, 59, 95, 158

D
desire, 3, 105, 150, 158
diaphragm, 146, 158
dumbbell, 30, 34, 36, 62–104, 158

E
epiphyseal plate, 7, 48, 149, 158
epiphysis, 7, 158

F
fast twitch, 25, 158
flexibility, 6, 52, 53, 117, 158
flexing, 18, 51, 158
force, 27, 117, 146–158
full range-of-motion, 42, 53, 75, 99, 158

G
guidelines, 4

H
hormones, 2, 27, 48, 146, 149, 158
hyperextension, 64, 88, 158

I
inhalation, 146, 158
interval sprints, 130, 158
in-season program, 11, 12, 48, 49, 158

J
joint, 2, 17, 59, 76, 94, 158

L
lactic acid, 24, 26, 42, 159
lean body mass, 145, 159
lifting belt, 5, 32, 71, 91, 92, 159
ligament, 1, 76, 159

M
major exercise, 60, 62–104, 131, 159
metabolism, 150, 159
motivation, 2, 3, 150, 159
motor unit, 24, 159
motor unit recruitment, 24, 159
muscle-bound, 1, 159
muscle fiber, 20, 24, 25, 43, 159
muscle tone, 24, 159
muscular endurance, 6, 24, 25, 43, 105, 108, 117, 129, 159

N
narrow stance, 62, 65, 159
nitrogen, 149, 159
NSCA, 14, 15, 155, 159

O
off-season program, 48, 49, 159
Olympic plates, 31, 159
Olympic set, 31, 159
one-hundred-ten pound set, 31, 159

overload, 26, 41, 42, 43, 159
overtraining, 41, 159

P
plyometrics, 117, 123, 159
poundage, 4, 159
power, 2, 6, 8, 11, 105, 107, 117, 123–126, 159
power lifting, 7, 12, 13, 15, 86, 87, 159
pro gain, 12, 145, 146, 159
progress chart, 43, 44–47, 52, 159
puberty, 2, 26, 48, 159

R
recovery, 41, 159
repetitions, 4, 42, 43, 48, 159
rest between sets, 43, 159
rest intervals, 24, 159

S
slow twitch, 25, 159
speed, 8, 13, 105, 117, 160
speed drills, 6, 41, 53, 106, 118–122, 132–143
split routine, 6, 40, 41, 48, 160
spotter, 4, 30, 62, 65, 67, 160
squat cage, 29, 30, 69, 71, 160
standard bar, 30, 31, 160
standard plates, 31, 160
strength, 6, 8, 11, 43, 160

strength training, 1, 6, 9, 10, 12, 13, 40, 41, 71, 145, 160
stretching routine, 30, 50, 52, 58, 160
stride frequency, 117, 160
stride length, 117, 160
supplementary exercise, 63–104, 160

T
techniques, 2, 59, 61–104, 117, 160
tendons, 1, 17, 18, 160
training goals, 3, 41, 106–110, 144, 150, 151, 160
training load, 42, 43, 160
training plateau, 41, 160
Tuflex, 4, 160

U
UPI (United Press International), 73, 101, 160
USFL (United States Football League), 148, 160

W
warm-up sets, 4, 52, 160
weight lifting, 7, 8, 9, 10, 12, 13, 15, 160
weight training, 2, 6, 160

Notes

If you have not purchased the Computerized Edition of DYNAMIC STRENGTH TRAINING FOR ATHLETES, but have now decided you would like to have the computer program, you may order the diskette (formatted to run on any Apple II series computer with at least 48K memory and 1 disk drive) with the order form below.

Programs included on the diskette:

- Exercise selection
- Progress input
- Record keeping

WM. C. BROWN PUBLISHERS
2460 Kerper Boulevard · P.O. Box 539
Dubuque, Iowa 52001

Please send me

___ DYNAMIC STRENGTH TRAINING
FOR ATHLETES DISKETTE
01251–4 $10.00

Name _____

Address _____

City _____

State _____ Zip _____

Phone: (_____)_____

Method of Payment
☐ Check/Money Order Enclosed (we'll pay shipping costs)
☐ Charge my account*
☐ VISA ☐ MASTER CHARGE
☐ AMERICAN EXPRESS

Account # ☐☐☐☐☐☐☐☐☐☐☐☐☐☐

MC Bank # ☐☐☐☐   Exp. Date _____

Signature _____
*(Add Shipping & Handling Costs $1.25)

Amount of Order .... $_____

Tax (CA, IA and LA Residents
add sales tax) .... $_____

Shipping/Handling .... $_____

TOTAL .... $_____